A Framework for

Continuing Education
for the
Health Professions

A FRAMEWORK FOR

CONTINUING EDUCATION FOR THE HEALTH PROFESSIONS

**With Application to Mental Health and
Mental Retardation/Developmental Disabilities
Administration**

STEPHEN M. SHORTELL, Ph.D.
Center for Health Services Research
Department of Health Services
School of Public Health and Community Medicine
University of Washington

Advisory Editors

JERRY O. ELDER, M.H.A.
Child Development and
Rehabilitation Center
University of Oregon Health Sciences Center

CHARLES V. KEERAN JR., M.S.W.
Neuropsychiatric Institute
University of California,
Los Angeles

ASSOCIATION OF UNIVERSITY PROGRAMS
AUPHA IN HEALTH ADMINISTRATION/WASHINGTON, D.C.

Library of Congress Cataloging in Publication Data

Shortell, Stephen M
   A framework for continuing education for the health professions.

   Bibliography: p. 55
   1. Mental health services—Administration—Study and teaching (Continuing education) I. Elder, Jerry O. II. Keeran, Charles V. III. Title.
IV. Title: Continuing education for the health professions.
RA790.8.S56   658'.91'36220715   78-4100
ISBN 0-914904-26-4

   Grateful appreciation is extended to the copyright owners for permission to use the following material:

   Edwin M. Bartee and Fred Cheyunski. "A Methodology for Process-Oriented Organizational Diagnosis." *The Journal of Applied Behavioral Science* 13 (1977) 53–68.

   Thomas Dolgoff. "Seminar in Mental Health Administration." Topeka, Kansas: The Menninger Foundation (unpublished).

   William Garove and Thomas Fernekes. "Overview: Management Training Program," Management Training Program, Center for Developmental and Learning Disorders, University of Alabama in Birmingham (unpublished).

   "Guidelines and Standards for Professional Master's Degree Programs in Public Affairs/Public Administration." Washington, D.C.: National Association of School of Public Affairs and Administration, 1974.

   M. S. Knowles. "Human Resources Development in DD." *Public Administration Review* 34 (March-April 1974) 117.

   "Management Issues Relevant to Mental Health Continuing Education." Western Interstate Commission on Higher Education. Conference, June 1975.

Published for the Association of University Programs in Health Administration by the Health Administration Press, School of Public Health, The University of Michigan

Contents

Preface

This monograph addresses the issue of continuing
education for administrators of mental health and
mental retardation/developmental disabilities (MH, MR/DD)[1]
facilities and programs. It describes some of the distinctive
characteristics of MH, MR/DD administration, discusses the
importance of continuing education for its practitioners, and
presents the various components of a quality continuing education program. Program organization, content, and implementation are described. Evaluation of program effectiveness
and the need for financial support and quality control are considered. Finally, specific recommendations are made for initi-
ating and implementing an effective continuing education program.

This publication is the collaborative product of a number
of organizations interested in continuing education for MH,
MR/DD administrators. In 1974, the Task Force on Mental
Health and Mental Retardation Administration (sponsored

[1] This report uses the following abbreviations: MH for *Mental Health*, MR for
Mental Retardation, and DD for *Developmental Disabilities*. The terms *mental retardation* and *developmental disabilities* are often combined into a single symbol,
MR/DD. It is used here to denote that our deliberations were intended to include all
mental retardation services while acknowledging that not all mentally retarded
persons are developmentally disabled. The entire phrase *mental health, mental retardation and developmental disabilities* is referred to as MH, MR/DD.

by the Association of Mental Health Administrators, the Association of University Programs in Health Administration, and the American Psychiatric Association) established a Continuing Education Committee, chaired by Charles V. Keeran, Jr. In the same year, the Administrator Section of the Association of University Affiliated Facilities (AUAF)[2] established its Project on Education for MR/DD Administrators, chaired by Jerry O. Elder.

Collaboration between the Committee and the Project on a number of related problems resulted in the establishment, in 1975, of a Joint Committee to consider continuing education for mental health and mental retardation/developmental disabilities administrators.

Specific efforts in this area evolved from concern regarding the ability of practicing administrators to function effectively in the dynamic MH, MR/DD fields. Since administrators in these fields are drawn from a variety of disciplines including psychiatry, administration, psychology, and social work, all bring to the position the knowledge and skills of a particular discipline; few bring the combined skills necessary for effective administration in these settings. Service practitioners have needed administrative skills while those with administrative experience have required information about client populations, types of intervention, the roles of service disciplines, and the family. Usually, the compensating knowledge and skills have been acquired through experience, independent study, and informal discussions. Members of the Joint Committee were convinced that improved administrative skills could be achieved more effectively by a structured and well-articulated continuing education program.

The Joint Committee first considered the similarities and differences between mental health administration and mental retardation/developmental disabilities administration. It

---

[2] *University Affiliated Facilities* (UAFs) refers to university-based and/or affiliated interdisciplinary training programs in mental retardation/developmental disabilities. However, in July, 1976, the AUAF was renamed the "Association of University Affiliated Programs" (AUAP) and will be referred to as such in other parts of this monograph.

concluded that the similarities are sufficient for a combined discussion of continuing education.[3] This conclusion is in no way intended to imply that differences do not exist, but rather that the differences do not seem sufficient to warrant entirely separate approaches to continuing education for administration.

Other issues considered by the Joint Committee before its development of a continuing education strategy were the appropriate academic locus for a continuing education program for MH, MR/DD administrators and whether MH, MR/DD administration is sufficiently different from health administration or human services administration to warrant a separate curriculum. The Committee concluded that competence to teach the concepts of administration should be the primary factor in determining the academic locus. In some schools this competence may be found in programs dealing with the MH, MR/DD fields, but more often than not it will be found in graduate schools of public administration, social welfare, public health, health administration, and management. Consequently, the Committee concluded that continuing education programs for the MH, MR/DD administrator should emphasize the principles of management and their application to MH, MR/DD administration.

With these two questions resolved, the Committee met to draft a table of contents and chapter outlines for a publication on continuing education for the MH, MR/DD administrator. The outlines drafted by the Committee were reviewed by the full membership of both the Task Force on Mental Health and Mental Retardation Administration, and the Administrator

---

[3] This is especially true when the MR/DD program is part of a health, or mental health, system. Dr. Phillip Roos (Executive Director of the National Association for Retarded Citizens, and a member of the Task Force on Mental Health and Mental Retardation Administration) cites major differences between independent MR/DD facilities and those which are part of a human service system other than health. The differences include methods of funding, philosophical assumptions, major techniques of intervention, and terminology. To illustrate the latter point, the human services-based MR/DD facilities use the terms *condition* and *client* rather than the *illness* and *patient* terminology of a health system-based MR/DD facility. This publication uses the former, more broadly-based terminology.

Section of the AUAF. Their recommendations were incorporated in the final outline.

A Maternal and Child Health grant from the Health Services Administration to the University Affiliated Facility at the University of Oregon's Health Sciences Center enabled the Committee to engage Stephen Shortell to provide staff support and to write the final report. Dr. Shortell's background and experience contributed significantly to the scope and depth of the Committee's deliberations and to the quality of the final document.

The draft and final manuscript prepared by Dr. Shortell were also reviewed by the full membership of both the Task Force and the Administrator Section of the AUAF. Their suggestions were incorporated in the final document, with Mr. Elder, Mr. Keeran, and Dr. Shortell serving as the final editorial board.

We hope that the text will be a significant contribution to the literature on continuing education for MH, MR/DD administrators. While the material presented is applied specifically to the administration of MH, MR/DD services, the framework may provide food for thought and be applicable to continuing education for other health professions. The Appendices, although not exhaustive, provide good examples of diverse approaches.

Jerry O. Elder
Charles V. Keeran, Jr.

Acknowledgments

We wish to express grateful appreciation for support provided by the following organizations and for the contribution by their members:

Task Force on Mental Health
and Mental Retardation Administration

JOHN R. MALBAN, *Chairman*
University of Minnesota

WALTER BARTON, M.D.
Veterans Administration General
  Hospital
White River Junction, Vermont

WILLIAM BYRON
State of New York
Department of Mental Hygiene

WILLIAM CAMPBELL
Glenwood State Hospital-School
Glenwood, Iowa

SAUL FELDMAN, D.P.A.
National Institute of Mental Health

BARRY GREEN, Ph.D.
Trinity University

PHILLIP B. HALLEN
Maurice Falk Medical Fund

GARY LLOYD, Ph.D.
University of Houston

Charles V. Keeran, Jr.
University of California, Los Angeles

Phillip Roos, Ph.D.
National Association for
  Retarded Citizens

Stanley Yolles M.D.
State University of New York,
Stony Brook

Continuing Education Committee

Charles V. Keeran, *Chairman*

William Byron
State of New York
Department of Mental Hygiene

Gary Lloyd, Ph.D.
University of Houton

Administrator Section
Association of University Affiliated Programs

Project on Education for
MR/DD Administrators

Jerry O. Elder, *Chairman*
University of Oregon

R. Wilburn Clouse
George Peabody College for Teachers

William Garove, Ph.D.
University of Alabama Medical Center

J. Robert Gray
University of North Carolina

Charles V. Keeran, Jr.
University of California, Los Angeles

Melvin D. Peters
University of Tennessee

Adrian E. Williamson
University of Colorado

We also wish to thank Patricia A. Cahill of the Association of University Programs in Health Administration for her help in preparing this manuscript.

Introduction

Assumptions and Guidelines

The approach to continuing education developed in this monograph is based on several assumptions and guidelines. Since this report is not intended to be all things to all people, it is useful to state these explicitly:

1. While recognizing that the administration of mental health and mental retardation/developmental disabilities (MH, MR/DD) services must be concerned with *all* of the human services, the primary focus of this report will be on the administrator's role vis-à-vis the *health services* delivery system. It is felt that one of the best ways in which the administrator of mental disability services can relate to the other human service systems (education, rehabilitation, corrections, social services, etc.) is by first having a thorough knowledge and understanding of the health services system and the role of management within that system.

2. There is enough similarity among mental health, mental retardation, and developmental disabilities administration to develop a meaningful generic approach to continuing education.

3. There is a great demand for higher quality managerial skills in MH, MR/DD administration. Since only a

small percentage of this demand will be met by forth-coming graduates of administration programs, quality continuing education programs must be developed for existing administrators.

4. While it is possible to devise a generic approach to continuing education of MH, MR/DD administrators, individual programs must be designed to serve their particular audience(s) and will vary according to:

   a) whether the audience consists primarily of mental health administrators or mental retardation/developmental disabilities administrators;

   b) whether the administrators have a clinical or a nonclinical background;

   c) the types of organizations in which the administrators are employed, e.g., whether in state mental health departments, community mental health agencies, or privately operated organizations;

   d) the size of the organization;

   e) the level at which the individual is employed in the organization.

5. In view of these contingencies, and the experience which the administrator brings to the learning environment, continuing education must be based on participation by the practitioner and the faculty member. (See, for example, Foley's discussion of the "andragogical model," 1975.) Administrators, their organizations, and faculty can contribute to each other's continuing education.

6. Although this monograph is addressed to MH, MR/DD continuing education efforts whether university-affiliated or otherwise, most of the examples focus on the university-based model. There are several reasons for this choice: to capitalize on university resources; to build a bridge between the university and the world of practice; and to further develop relationships between MH, MR/DD continuing education and university-based graduate programs in business administration, public administration, and health services administration.

7. No recommendation is made regarding the appropriateness of particular units of the university (nor of the university itself) as the location for MH, MR/DD continuing education. The choice should be made on the basis of the type of courses to be taught, the nature of the clientele involved, and most importantly, on the relative strengths, weaknesses, and interests of the university units and non–university-related continuing education agencies in the area.

8. *Continuing education efforts must be continually evaluated* with regard to the quality of the applicant to the program, the quality of the organization responsible for the program, and the quality and nature of the changes (if any) effected by the program (i.e., impact evaluation).

9. In view of the need for improved managerial skills, this is intended to be an active–user-oriented report. It is expected that the following groups will find the report to be a useful guide for the development of continuing education policies and programs:

   a) committees of national organizations, such as the Association of University Programs in Health Administration (AUPHA), Association of Mental Health Administrators (AMHA), American Psychiatric Association (APA), Association of Private Psychiatric Facilities (APPF), the National Association of State Mental Health Program Directors (NASM-HPD), the American Hospital Association's Psychiatric Services Section, Association of University Affiliated Programs (AUAP), American Society of Public Administrators (ASPA), American Public Health Association (APHA), Western Interstate Commission on Higher Education (WICHE), and Southern Regional Educational Board (SREB), in their program planning activities;

   b) universities—in developing continuing education programs;

   c) agencies responsible for planning and public

policy development and those providing re-sources for funding;

d) for continuing education efforts in other fields such as health services, nursing home, and ambulatory care administration.

In sum, this is intended to be a working document to serve as a focus for discussion and debate and from which particular actions may be taken to increase the quality of continuing education efforts in MH, MR/DD administration.

I

The Nature of Mental Health
and Mental Retardation/Developmental
Disabilities Administration

The Importance of Administration

The delivery of health services has become increasingly complex. Changes in medical technology, social norms, and legal definitions of "illness"; the expanding role of federal and state governments in financing and delivering services; and rising expectations and demands for accountability to the public have interacted to produce unprecedented uncertainties for health care professionals.

For a variety of reasons (well documented at the First National Conference on Education for Mental Health Administration), the delivery of mental health and mental retardation/developmental disabilities (MH, MR/DD) services has been particularly affected by such changes—changes which have revealed a relative lack of trained, sophisticated management to cope with the myriad forces. While poor management may remain inconspicuous in a simple environment, the stresses and strains of change render it embarrassingly evident.

The movement toward the de-institutionalization of mental health patients further highlights the need for better adminis-

1

tration. It places greater demands upon administration to assess the supply of community-based mental health services, to educate the local community, and to establish the necessary coordination and communication among agencies. These activities require the skills and understanding of planning methodologies, community politics, strategies for change, and interorganizational relationships. Administrators possessing such skills and understanding are likely to be better able to cope with the complexities inherent in the de-institutionalization process.

The need for better prepared MH, MR/DD administrators is widely acknowledged. (See, for example, Perspectives on Mental Health and Mental Retardation Administration, 1975.) Issues concerning their recruitment, selection, and graduate education have been discussed in a previous report, *Education of Health Services Administrators in an Interdisciplinary Model* (J. Elder et al., 1976). The objective of the present monograph is to involve academic and professional groups in a discussion of the *continuing* education needs of MH, MR/DD administrators and to promote behavior which will increase the number and quality of continuing education opportunities.

The Nature of MH, MR/DD Administration

To provide a framework for developing models of continuing education, it is necessary to understand the nature of the administrative task. Thompson (1967) defines administration as "shooting at a moving target." While seemingly glib and cryptic, this definition holds several important implications. Thompson stresses the administrator's ability to maintain the organization's effectiveness and influence amidst a variety of changing forces and circumstances. In somewhat more concrete terms, Thompson's definition involves the administrator's ability to co-align or *configurate* (Shortell, 1976) the organization's internal structure and processes to fit best the nature and demands of the external environment. It is Thompson's contention, supported by some of the empirical literature (Lawrence and Lorsch, 1967; Becker and Neuhauser, 1975),

2

that organizations whose internal designs are better matched with the nature of their task and with their external environment demonstrate greater efficiency and deliver a higher quality of services.

The notion of co-alignment emphasizes the administrator's role as technician, politician, and visionary. To implement change successfully and to provide effective day-to-day operation, the administrator must possess, and be able to apply, certain basic, technical skills in financial management, personnel administration, and information systems. To negotiate with the external environment, the administrator needs certain "political" skills relevant to community organization and politics, and to inter-organizational relationships. To detect the need for change, the administrator must develop an ability to survey the environment with a view to anticipating new developments and creating new opportunities for his or her organization. Continuing education programs should contribute not only to the development of administrators' technical and political skills and knowledge, but also to their visionary capabilities. For example, delphi and nominal group decision-making techniques are examples of approaches to helping individuals think in futuristic terms, to assessing the implications of alternatives, and to assigning priorities.

Defining administration as "shooting at a moving target" is appropriate for continuing education discussions in general, and particularly for the continuing education of MH, MR/DD administrators. In the most naive sense, if administration did not involve continuous change (the moving target) there would be little need for continuing education of any kind. Management theory and skills could be taught in graduate school and graduates sent out with their tool kit and certificates as "expert marksmen"; the most that would be needed might be periodic refresher courses. The volatility of the health services environment has led to an increased demand for continuing education courses of many sorts. This is particularly true regarding MH, MR/DD services, due to the nature of the services and to the relative lack of formal management preparation of many administrators of these services.

The administration of MH, MR/DD services has much in common with other types of health services administration but also exhibits differences which hold important implications for the development of continuing education programs. Feldman (1973) has outlined some of these distinguishing characteristics:

1. heavy reliance on public funding and governmental control
2. close involvement with a wide range of professionals who have high needs for autonomy
3. a highly personal therapist-client relationship
4. a highly dependent client population
5. a client population with which it is frequently difficult to relate therapeutically
6. a highly intangible product for which criteria of success are difficult to establish
7. a clientele whose condition carries considerable social stigma

To the above might be added the following characteristics, outlined in *Education of Health Services Administrators in an Interdisciplinary Model*:

8. an early age of entry into the system, particularly among mentally retarded and mentally disabled children
9. unusually complex legal issues due to the impaired judgment of some clients, particularly the mentally retarded and disabled
10. the chronicity of the condition involved—the length of time for which the individual requires services
11. the strong involvement of consumers
12. the need for links with other service systems (education, vocational rehabilitation, religious institutions, etc.)

The last three items are of particular concern to the administrator of MR/DD services.

Perhaps the most important difference between MH, MR/

4

DD administration and other forms of health services administration (such as hospital administration, ambulatory care administration, and nursing home administration) involves *the more extended network of external environmental relationships which must be maintained.* This is further complicated by the existence of both clinical and nonclinical routes to administrative positions in the delivery of MH, MR/DD services—in contrast to the predominantly nonclinical route to hospital, ambulatory care, and nursing home administration. The MH, MR/DD audience for continuing education is a heterogeneous group which finds itself involved in the administration of highly personal services for individuals who require a broad array of services and special considerations. These circumstances place additional demands on management skills and require the development of an approach to continuing education which realistically recognizes the nature of the environment in which administrators of MH, MR/DD services practice.

II

Philosophy and Approach to Continuing Education For Administrators of Mental Health and Mental Retardation/Developmental Disabilities Services

Working Definition of Continuing Education

Broadly defined, continuing education for administrators of mental health and mental retardation/developmental disabilities (MH, MR/DD) services could include any educational activity through which *systematic* learning opportunities are provided, including formal and informal courses, conferences, conventions, symposia, seminars, institutes, and workshops. In an even broader sense, any daily experience from which an individual is able to obtain a new skill, a new idea, or a new insight which can be generalized to future situations can be considered continuing education. In defining continuing education in somewhat more circumscribed terms, this report does not question the obvious value of a broad view of continuing education. Rather, it reflects the need to develop a working definition of continuing education upon which specific programs and activities can be built.

We define continuing education as *the planned learning,*

beyond the basic professional education, of generic administrative and management skills relevant to the delivery of MH, MR/DD services. Planned learning refers to learning oriented to stated objectives, and to the evaluation of both the process and outcome of the learning experience. *Generic administrative and management skills* are those which can be applied to a wide variety of situations which the MH, MR/DD administrator will face in his or her career. Although valuable, purely informational programs designed to bring practitioners up-to-date (for example, on the latest legislation in the field or the latest funding developments in Washington) would not constitute continuing education as we have defined it. Continuing education must be relevant to today's problem but must also transcend it. The definition of administration as "shooting at a moving target" reflects the reality that the problems of today are not the problems of tomorrow; consequently, we emphasize the development of generic skills, knowledge, and value orientations which can be useful to the administrator in a variety of circumstances.

The differences between this concept of continuing education and in-service education should also be mentioned. The principal distinctions are outlined in Figure II-1. Figure II-1 presents "ideal" distinctions and is not meant to suggest that these prevail in all situations, nor that meaningful continuing education programs cannot be conducted on an in-service basis. Rather, the two most important distinctions lie in the extent to which formal standards and evaluation practices exist, and the extent to which the learning involved is of a generic rather than a specific nature. Formal standards and evaluations refer to the extent to which criteria are established for entry into the program, the extent to which content and instructional standards exist, and the extent to which standards are developed for evaluating the process and outcome of the learning experience. From an employing organization's standpoint, the concept of generic versus specific training is central to the economics of investment in human capital (Schultz, 1962; Becker, 1964). In brief, it is usually more "profitable" for an organization to provide "specific training"

7

FIGURE II–1

Primary Distinctions between Continuing Education and In-Service Education

Continuing Education	In-Service Education
1. May be either in-house or outside the organization, usually the latter	1. Usually in-house
2. Has formal standards and evaluation, either university-, professional association-, or agency-based	2. Standards and evaluation often informal or nonexistent
3. Is more oriented toward development of individuals' abilities which can cut across organizations and varying situations; that is, *generic* training	3. Oriented toward present organization and problems; that is, *specific* training

which will help solve immediate day-to-day problems and be directly relevant to the organization's interest than to provide educational experiences of a more general nature which may serve mainly to increase the individual's attractiveness to other organizations. This may partially explain why in-service education programs tend to be relatively narrowly focused and why it is necessary to go outside a given organization for continuing education programs of a more substantive and generic nature.

Finally, we restrict our working definition of continuing education primarily to the part-time education of individuals concurrently employed in a delivery organization. Technically, this would also include part-time students pursuing an advanced degree over a prolonged period of time and would encompass extended university programs as well. However, since a relatively small percentage of individuals in the field is in either of these situations, and since they are not generally perceived as major alternatives for large numbers of practicing administrators, little attention will be given to them in this report.

The above restriction might also eliminate mid-career fellowship and traineeship programs, in which an individual has left an organization or is on an extended leave of absence. Again, our intention is not to exclude these activities from the broad umbrella of continuing education activities which might be undertaken by those interested in furthering the quality of management in MH, MR/DD administration; nevertheless, this report will not deal in depth with the content of such programs.

In summary, we define continuing education as a program of structured, planned learning experiences designed for practicing administrators of MH, MR/DD programs, with the objectives of increasing generic managerial skills and knowledge and exploring the implications of different value orientations. The learning experiences may or may not be university-based and, as will be discussed in Chapters III and IV, they may take a number of different approaches and formats.

A Conceptual Model of Continuing Education

Having outlined some basic assumptions and provided a working definition of continuing education, it is possible to develop a general framework for thinking about the process of continuing education for MH, MR/DD administrators. The framework presented here is that of an *open systems approach* (von Bertalanffy, 1968; Katz and Kahn, 1966), *which places a high value on responsiveness to new opportunities and adaptation to changing circumstances.* Although the open systems approach is neither the only approach nor necessarily the best approach for addressing the issues at hand, it does include several key ideas relevant to the dynamic nature of MH, MR/DD administration as reflected in the earlier definition of administration as "shooting at a moving target."

For example, an open systems approach makes it possible to examine the relationship among the inputs into the educational process, the actual use of these inputs in the educational experience (i.e., the transformation process), and the outputs produced. There are then three principal components to consider in developing further continuing education opportunities for the field: inputs and inflows; the transformation process; and outputs. *Inputs* and *inflows* refer to the acquisition of resources which will be used in the educational process. An input is distinguished from an inflow in that an input is transformed into an output; that is, the original state of the input is altered. Examples include the resources brought to the educational experience by the "participant/administrator" (e.g., experience, knowledge, and skills); faculty resources and abilities; and resources of the employing organization. In contrast, inflows represent resources (e.g., facilities, equipment, and supplies) which are used in the educational process but which are not transformed into outputs. They may be expended in the process of producing outputs (and in that sense may be "altered") but they do not assume a new form or take on an added dimension.

The *transformation process* refers to the various strategies of mixing inputs and inflows to produce outputs; the outputs, in this case, are additions to the managerial skill and knowledge base of administrators of mental disability services. In concrete terms, the focus is on issues of curriculum content, teaching and learning methodologies, and the interaction which occurs among faculty and participant/administrators.

As suggested above, the *outputs* are a function of the transformation process and, in the current context, comprise the acquisition of additional managerial knowledge, skill, and value orientations. This, of course, requires evaluation and evaluation leads to feedback, which makes the continuing education process (like all open systems) dynamic and responsive to change. An overview of the open systems approach is presented in Figure II-2.

There are several advantages to viewing continuing education in an open systems framework. The first is that it emphasizes the *interdependence of continuing education activities.* The extent to which management expertise can be improved depends upon the quality of the human and technological resources available (inputs and inflows) and the nature of the educational (transformation) process. In turn, the extent to which a continuing education activity is able to prosper depends upon the ability to evaluate the outputs, to communicate the information to relevant parties, and to *act upon* the information.

A second advantage of this perspective is that it emphasizes the dynamic nature of continuing education activities. Forces are in continuous motion, not unlike the environment in which MH, MR/DD administrators practice. The educational process itself thus reflects attributes of the world of practice, and learning becomes experiential as well as cognitive, leading to a greater probability that what is learned will be transferred to the operational setting.

FIGURE II–2

Open Systems Framework for Continuing Education

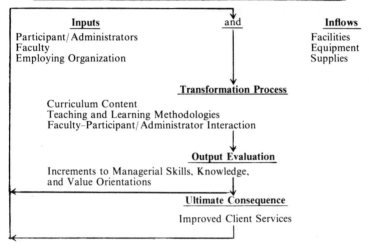

A third major advantage of the open systems perspective is that it emphasizes the principles of *equifinality* and *multi-finality*. The principle of *equifinality* states that *there are a variety of ways of reaching the same goal*. The principle of *multifinality* suggests that *similar inputs may lead to different outputs, and that similar initial conditions may lead to dis-similar end states*. The principle of equifinality emphasizes the need for *flexibility* in the development of continuing education programs for MH, MR/DD administrators. Several different approaches may be equally effective. The principle of multi-finality emphasizes the need for competent administration and organization of the continuing education program. Thus, two or more similar approaches with similar inputs and inflows

11

may result in varying levels of effectiveness depending on the quality of administration and faculty and the nature of the clientele involved.

For the reasons stated above, we feel an open systems framework is useful for conceptualizing the continuing education process and for developing continuing education programs and activities. For those involved in the development of such programs, it provides a conceptual map from which operational planning and implementation may proceed.

In this report our primary focus will be on the transformation process (curriculum content, etc.) and the outputs produced (additions to management skill, etc.) but, in using an open systems approach, we will inevitably comment on inputs and inflows as well.

III

The Curriculum:
Organization and Content

Assessment of Needs

The development of curriculum content must be based on a careful assessment of the needs of practicing administrators. Various groups and conferences over the past several years have outlined the managerial implications of the changing characteristics of mental health and mental retardation/developmental disabilities (MH, MR/DD) administration noted in Chapter I. A list of such implications would include the need for:

1. designing more effective organizational structures to deal with a rapidly changing environment;
2. improved techniques of managerial planning and control, e.g., MBO and PERT;
3. greater commitment to, and development of, skills in program evaluation;
4. greater exposure to the tools of cost accounting and financial management;
5. greater understanding of small group dynamics, interpersonal behavior, leadership styles, and communications processes;

6. additional training in strategies of coordinating work and decision making;
7. greater sensitivity to community groups, political networks, and inter-organizational relationships, and the development of strategies for working with them; and
8. a greater understanding of the managerial implications of legal and technological changes in the definition of illness and methodologies available for treatment.

While these are among the most important areas which need to be addressed regarding continuing education programs, it would be unwise for any university or agency to proceed without a careful assessment of the particular needs of administrators in its own geographical area. Several outstanding examples of needs assessment methodologies are available, including that employed by the Mental Health Administration Continuing Education Project at Tulane University (1975), and a process-oriented approach used by the Community Mental Health Management Development Program at Vanderbilt University (Bartee and Cheyunski, 1977). A description of the latter approach is provided in Appendix A.

Needs are obviously determined by many factors, but from a program development viewpoint the most important are: (1) the background of the administrator (i.e., clinical vs. nonclinical); (2) the type of organization at which the individual is employed; (3) the stage of the individual's career; and (4) the level at which the individual is employed. For example, in regard to background, an administrator with a primarily clinical background may express greater need for additional training in financial management and budgeting, while an administrator with a nonclinical background may express greater interest in developing interpersonal and small-group skills to deal with multi-disciplinary health care teams. Regarding the type of organization involved, directors of state residential care facilities may express a primary interest in the development of better internal management and control techniques, while community mental health center administrators, or administrators of developmental disability programs, may be more interested in courses dealing with community politics, consumer involvement, and inter-organizational relationships. In regard to stage of career and level in the organization, those occupying top management positions may express a greater need for expertise in dealing with outside parties and funding sources, while those at the middle management level may express a greater need for additional supervisory, program implementation, and evaluation skills. None of these contingencies negates the fact that all administrators need a thorough grounding in the fundamentals of organization theory and behavior and management practices. Rather, the above contingencies underscore the need for flexibility and practitioner involvement in program design.

Matrix Approaches

Once needs have been identified, it is possible to identify potentially relevant topics and disciplines. It is in this area that continuing education program staff and university faculty can be of assistance. Matrices can be devised which list needs or issues on one axis and the potentially relevant topics and disciplines on the other axis. *The advantage of the matrix approach is that it provides continuing education participants (both faculty and practitioners) with an overview of the disciplines and knowledge bases relevant for specific learning objectives.* The matrix approach is, of course, only one way of viewing curriculum issues. We present it simply to illustrate its general utility and flexibility, and recognize that other conceptualizations may be more appropriate in other situations. Several examples serve to illustrate the potential of the matrix approach.

Figure III-1 presents a matrix in which the general needs of MH, MR/DD administration identified earlier are presented on the y axis and various academic disciplines and knowledge areas are presented on the x axis. Several characteristics of this matrix should be noted. First, in no case does a need or issue require input from only one discipline or knowledge area. For example, in the case of multi-disciplinary professional

15

teams, course content must be drawn from organization theory, organization development, small-group theory, psychology, and sociology. The implication for university-based continuing education programs is a departure from the traditional graduate education organized around discrete courses in specific areas (for example, a course in organization theory followed by courses in organization development and community politics). In the world of practice, problems do not come one at a time or in such sequential fashion, and the busy administrator often does not have time to take a series of sequenced courses. Therefore, a single course must provide the most useful insights available from a number of different knowledge areas and present them in a fashion which facilitates integrative learning. If there is a need to improve the management of professional teams, some of the theoretical and empirical studies of the socialization of professionals should be integrated with: the psychology of perception and motivation; studies of small-group performance (concerned with varying leadership styles and types of participation); and team-building and organization design strategies (from organization development and organization theory). This is likely to require major changes in the habits of university faculty accustomed to teaching specialized courses, with less attention to integration of course material or the overall learning experience. (The exceptions, of course, are capstone courses, or small seminars, explicitly designed to provide integrative frameworks.) Thus, the development of continuing education courses for MH, MR/DD administrators will require a reorganization of existing faculty resources and different teaching strategies (e.g., team teaching), and greater involvement of practitioners in the educational process. In a word, the emphasis is on eclecticism in course content and methodology.

A second characteristic of the matrix shown in Figure III–1 is that it presents issues and knowledge areas at a fairly abstract level. While this is appropriate for providing an overview of continuing education needs, it may be less useful for designing courses to meet the needs. The needs and issues

FIGURE III-1

Matrix Approach I to Curriculum Organization for Continuing Education for MH, MR/DD Administration

Disciplines and Applied Knowledge Areas

General Needs and Issues	Cost Accounting	Public Finance	Program Evaluation	Organization Theory	Organization Development	Small-Group Theory	Political Science	Psychology	Sociology	Community Politics	Law	Economics
Organization Structures for Dealing with Changing Environments				X	X		X			X		X
Planning and Control	X	X	X									
Acquiring and Managing Financial Resources	X	X										X
Dealing with Multi-Disciplinary Professional Teams				X	X	X		X	X			
Work Coordination and Decision Making				X	X	X	X	X	X			X
Dealing with Community Groups and Outside Agencies				X	X		X	X	X	X		
Managing the Implications of Legal and Technological Change				X	X	X					X	
Other												

can, however, be listed at varying levels of concreteness (e.g., specific administrative functions, skills, and delivery system goals). Similarly, potential course content need not be grouped according to basic disciplines but can be organized according to applied knowledge areas such as "capital budgeting" or "wage and salary administration." Figure III-2 shows a matrix in which the disciplines and knowledge areas remain essentially the same as in Figure III-1 while the MH, MR/DD administration issues have been given a more specific *problem-oriented* focus.

Figure III-3 shows a third matrix in which *management functions* are identified on the *y* axis and academic disciplines and knowledge areas on the *x* axis. Figure III-3 also serves as an example of a matrix approach for developing content for a specific course. The functions listed in Figure III-3 are classic examples of management functions discussed in basic texts, around which a specific course in administrative theory and practice could be developed. Such a course (depending on its scope) would draw upon many, if not all, of the disciplines listed across the top of the matrix. An example of such a course, taught by Thomas Dolgoff at the Menninger Foundation, is shown in Appendix B.

We have not attempted to establish priorities regarding the content of MH, MR/DD continuing education in view of its many contingencies. However, we believe all MH, MR/DD administrators should have some basic skill in and understanding of management theory, organization design and interorganizational relationships; financial management and the budgetary process; and personnel administration (including wage and salary administration) and interpersonal and small-group relationships. Basic and advanced treatment of these areas would be most beneficial to MH, MR/DD administrators today, because they are at the heart of *public accountability*. Courses in these areas should address such issues as: (1) how to design an organization which will provide high quality services; (2) types of managerial practices which promote high quality; (3) how to acquire, allocate, and control the human and non-human resources which promote superior perform-

FIGURE III–2

Matrix Approach II to Curriculum Organization for
Continuing Education for MH, MR/DD Administration

Problem or Issue	Public Finance	Cost Accounting	Small-Group Theory	Organization Theory, Organization Development	Overview of Clinical Practice	Community Politics	Labor Relations	Political Science
Establishing Cost Centers	X	X						
Dealing with Multiple Funding Sources	X			X		X		X
Working with Multi-Disciplinary Health Care Teams			X	X	X			
Establishing Policy Regarding De-institutionalization				X	X	X		X
Dealing with Labor Unions, Etc.			X				X	

19

ance; and (4) how to provide the motivation, communication, and conflict resolution strategies necessary for superior performance.

In summary, it should be emphasized that there are many ways of thinking about continuing education curriculum content. The matrix concept presented here is only one such approach. Several examples have been provided, however, to indicate its potential usefulness and adaptability. But regardless of the particular approach used, the emphasis should be on *substantive generic learning*, which has utility beyond "today's problem," and on the *application of basic disciplinary knowledge to the MH, MR/DD administrative setting.* A third principle, which follows from the above two, is the need for reinforcement. This will be discussed in further detail in Chapter IV.

Evaluation

Evaluating any program (or course) is deceptively difficult, because despite the best intentions, the evaluation process is usually more difficult than even the most somber pessimist would predict. In an open systems approach to continuing education feedback is essential to improvement, and feedback is dependent upon evaluation of current activities. A recent survey conducted by the Western Center for Continuing Education in Mental Health (Bloom, 1974) revealed that "evaluating the impact of participation in CE [Continuing Education] programs on subsequent . . . administrative performance" was one of the three most important issues.

Traditionally, the evaluation of continuing education programs has been little more than the study of the amount of effort expended. More recently, attempts have been made to conduct what might be called *intermediate outcome* evaluations in which participants are asked to evaluate what they have learned and to what extent learning objectives have been met. In some courses needs assessment questionnaires are distributed, and particular behavioral learning objectives are developed from the results. Upon completion of the course,

FIGURE III-3

Matrix Approach III to Curriculum Organization for Continuing Education for MH, MR/DD Administration

Functions of Management	Psychology (Individual Behavior)	Sociology and Social Psychology (Group Behavior)	Decision Theory (Rational Choice)	Mathematics Operations Research (Systems Theory)	Practice (Management Experience)
PLANNING					
Being Aware of Opportunity					Budgeting
Establishing Objectives	Management by objectives	Nominal group technique			
Forecasting				Delphi technique	
Decision Making	X				
Determining Alternative Courses	X			Simulation	
Evaluating Alternative Courses	X		Decision trees		
Selecting a Course			Expected utility, subjective probability	Queuing theory, linear programming	
Other					

FIGURE III-3

Matrix Approach III to Curriculum Organization for Continuing Education for MH, MR/DD Administration

Functions of Management	Psychology (Individual Behavior)	Sociology and Social Psychology (Group Behavior)	Decision Theory (Rational Choice)	Mathematics Operations Research (Systems Theory)	Practice (Management) Experience
ORGANIZING					
Span of Management	Management by objectives	Nominal group technique			
Departmentalization	X	X			
Assignment of Activities	X	X			
Line and Staff Authority	X	X			
Service Departments	X	X			
Decentralization of Authority	X	X			
Committees	X	X			
Other					
STAFFING					
Selection of Staff	Performance review and evaluation	Task differentiation and specialization			Task differentiation and specialization
Appraisal of Staff	X				
Assignment of Staff					
Development and Training of Staff		X		Linear programming	

	Performance review and evaluation	Task differentiation and specialization		Management information systems / Cybernetic theory / Program budgeting, PERT (CPM)	Financial statements
DIRECTING					
Motivation	X				
Communication	T-groups, (lab training)	X			
Leadership		X			
Other					
CONTROLLING					
Feedback Process	Performance review and evaluation				
Special Control Techniques				Management information systems	
				Cybernetic theory	
				Program budgeting, PERT (CPM)	
Control of Overall Performance					Financial statements
Other					

faculty and students assess the extent to which the objectives have been met. An example, developed by the National Association of Schools of Public Affairs and Administration (1974) is provided in Appendix C.

While intermediate outcome evaluations can be extremely valuable, many prefer *impact evaluation*, which is designed to assess the effects of continuing education on administrative behavior in the organizational setting. Interest in impact evaluations is understandable since it is the actual behavior of administrators that is of greatest consequence to an organization. But, if other types of evaluations seem difficult to perform, impact evaluations often appear nearly impossible. This is due to a number of factors including: exposure of only a single individual or at most a few individuals from the same organization to the continuing education program; the vast number of variables which affect administrative behavior and organizational performance; and the difficulty of measuring even the more important variables, particularly in terms of the administrative and political problems involved in attempting such designs.

Despite the difficulties involved, it is essential that *every continuing education effort be evaluated in a way that will yield information useful for further improvement*. While, in the beginning stages of a program, process-oriented and intermediate outcome evaluations may prove most useful, in the long run the most valuable information is likely to come from impact evaluations. One example of the latter is the administration, before and after a continuing education program, of the *Styles of Management Inventory* (Blake and Mouton, 1964). This instrument is designed to obtain individuals' perceptions of behavioral change and could be administered to the administrator who participated in the program and to his supervisors, peers, and subordinates. Another approach is to identify several salient, highly visible decision events (e.g., hiring or firing a key employee, adding or deleting a service, or staying within a budget) and to compare the administrator's performance before and after the program. Although the decision events would never be identical, the focus would be on

24

the extent to which the administrator used skills, knowledge, and insights gained from the program.

The costs of conducting various types of evaluation must always be kept in mind. In general, impact evaluation is more costly than process evaluation. Estimates from the evaluation of continuing medical education programs indicate that participant evaluation can be obtained for about 2 percent of the course's cost, a pretest and post-test for about 6 percent, a mail survey of performance change for 113 percent, and a combination of survey and direct observation of behavior change for 371 percent ("Costs of Evaluation," 1970).

Greater documentation and sharing of information regarding evaluation efforts by continuing educators in MH, MR/DD administration is needed, so that useful guidelines and estimates can be developed in this field.

The evaluation of continuing education programs is a major challenge to those interested in improving the quality of MH, MR/DD administration. Quasi-experimental evaluations (Campbell and Stanley, 1966; Shortell and Richardson, 1978), such as those noted above, need to be further explored. Consideration should also be given to such approaches as the multiple-time series design, interrupted time series design, before-and-after matched samples design, and various "patched up" designs (such as comparing the performance of a group of administrators which has undergone the program with that of a group ready to begin it). These approaches deserve much greater attention from continuing education directors than they have received to date.

IV

The Curriculum:
Implementation Strategies
and Learning Methodologies

While the last chapter was primarily concerned with issues of content, the focus of this chapter is on issues of process, such as the location of programs, faculty staffing, teaching and learning methodologies, funding, and providing for program continuity.

Location

Continuing education programs may be conducted in a variety of settings, and under a variety of sponsors, including colleges and universities and organizations affiliated with them (e.g., the Western Interstate Commission on Higher Education); professional associations (e.g., the American Psychiatric Association or the Association of Mental Health Administrators); and educational organizations—such as the University Affiliated Programs (UAPs). The actual setting or sponsorship is less important than that the following two principles be followed: (1) course content must be focused on the needs of the field; and (2) there must be involvement with ongoing delivery settings.

Perhaps the most apparent distinction is that between university-based or affiliated programs and non-university-based programs. The strength of the university-based or affiliated programs appears to be in the communication of material which requires a deductive approach—an approach which proceeds from the general to the particular. The advantage of the non-university-based setting seems to lie in the communication of material which requires an inductive approach—proceeding from particular situations and circumstances to the formulation of general principles. This distinction is somewhat artificial since an effective continuing education program must use both approaches. While most of the subsequent discussion will focus primarily on university-based or affiliated programs, we believe the ideas developed are also generally applicable to non-university-based programs.

There is no single "best" place within the university for continuing education programs. Successful programs can be developed equally well in, e.g., schools of public affairs, social work, business administration, public health, departments of psychiatry and related areas. The continuing education program should capitalize on the strengths of particular departments and schools in the university. It is also important that duplication of course work be avoided; in some cases, collaboration among departments or schools may be the best approach.

If the continuing education program is university-based or affiliated, the comparative advantages of on-campus versus off-campus courses should be considered. The primary advantages of on-campus courses include the proximity of university resources (e.g., libraries and faculty) and the opportunity for the practitioner to get away from daily pressures and problems. The primary advantages of the off-campus setting include its greater proximity to practitioners (particularly to those in rural areas) and the opportunity for university-based faculty to experience the problems and issues existing within the organizational setting.

The potential of these advantages will, of course, be affected by such factors as the nature of the course and the back-

28

grounds of the participants. For example, a course focusing on a relatively self-contained topic such as capital budgeting might well be able to be presented off-campus, while a course focusing on policy formulation and implementation might be more appropriately conducted on-campus.

If the class consists primarily of individuals from a single agency, it may be best to conduct the course off-campus, at the agency; for a class composed of individuals from a number of different organizations, it may be more advantageous to meet on-campus. In many cases, a combination of off-campus and on-campus activities will be required. This is particularly true for programs which continue for several months, and for programs offered to rural audiences. The University of Alabama's Management Training Program (Garove, 1975) and the University of Missouri's continuing education program (Boissoneau, 1975) are excellent examples of combined on-campus and off-campus activities—complemented by correspondence course work and telephone networks.

Faculty Considerations

Since faculty and practitioners are the most important resources in the continuing education process, the potential for improved mental health and mental retardation/developmental disabilities (MH, MR/DD) administration depends on what these two groups learn from each other. The university-based faculty involved in continuing education should be of the same quality as that available to full-time students. To ensure such quality, equal recognition (regarding promotion criteria, salary increases, etc.) must be given to faculty participation in continuing education. Appropriately, all full-time faculty of the University of Chicago's Graduate School of Business are required to teach in its evening program for part-time students.

It is essential that the university-based faculty be sufficiently familiar with MH, MR/DD administration in order to adapt their material to the needs of practicing administrators. Although this is not easily accomplished, several strategies are available, including: work/study exchanges between university faculty and MH, MR/DD personnel; consultation and technical assistance activities with MH, MR/DD agencies; and applied managerial and organizational research involving university faculty and MH, MR/DD administrators.

It is important to note the contribution which practicing administrators can make to continuing education. A course conducted by a university-based faculty member and a practicing administrator can be a particularly valuable experience and can increase the likelihood that what is learned in the classroom will be applied in practice.

Teaching and Learning Methodologies

Continuing education programs should capitalize on the experience and insights of the practitioner. There should be more experimentation with "adult-centered" approaches to learning (Knowles, 1974; Dolgoff, 1975; Foley, 1975; Argyris and Schon, 1974) without necessarily completely abandoning the pedagogical techniques which have frequently proven useful with less experienced individuals. The primary difference between adult-centered learning and pedagogy lies in the difference between active and passive learning. The major differences in assumptions and processes are summarized in Figure IV-1. It should be noted that these are somewhat over-stated in order to emphasize the basic distinctions.

The *need for reinforcement* is a key issue in the continuing education of MH, MR/DD administrators. Whenever possible, there should be on-the-job application of what is learned in the educational setting. In the survey of mental health continuing educators cited earlier (Bloom, 1974), "increasing the likelihood that participants in continuing education programs will have the opportunity to implement what they have learned" was rated among the areas of greatest importance. Because adult-centered learning emphasizes active learning and draws upon the individual's work experience, it seems most conducive to the successful transfer and application of new knowledge, skills, and value formations into the operational setting.

30

FIGURE IV-1

Differences in Assumptions and Process Elements: Pedagogy versus Andragogy

Assumptions

	Pedagogy	Andragogy
Self-Concept	Dependency	Increasing self-directiveness
Experience	Of little worth	Learners are a rich resource for learning
Readiness	Biological development Social pressure	Developmental tasks of social roles
Time perspective	Postponed application	Immediacy of application
Orientation to learning	Subject centered	Problem centered

Process Elements

	Pedagogy	Andragogy
Climate	Authority-oriented Formal Competitive	Mutuality Respectful Collaborative Informal
Planning	By teacher	Mechanism for mutual planning
Diagnosis of needs	By teacher	Mutual self-diagnosis
Formulation of objectives	By teacher	Mutual negotiation
Design	Logic of the subject matter Content units	Sequenced in terms of readiness problem units
Activities	Transmittal techniques	Experiential techniques (inquiry)
Evaluation	By teacher	Mutual rediagnosis of needs Mutual measurement of program

Source: M. S. Knowles, "Human Resources Development in OD," *Public Administration Review* 34 (March/April 1974), 117. Reprinted by permission of *Public Administration Review*.

Continuing education programs developed at Harvard, Vanderbilt, and Alabama serve as examples of the adult-centered learning approach and learning reinforcement strategies. The Harvard Medical School's Continuing Education Program for Mental Health Planners and Administrators (Caplan, 1974) offers six three-day seminars during a two-year period in which participants have the opportunity to apply new skills and knowledge in their work situations and to bring job-related issues back to the learning setting. Case materials are developed based on the participants' administrative experiences. The seminars address issues related to administrative principles, policy development, planning methods, program models, manpower utilization, and program evaluation.

Funded by the Tennessee Department of Mental Health, Vanderbilt University is developing a Community Mental Health Management Development Program. This program is based on the principle that management learning experiences must be based on the problem area itself, as perceived by practicing administrators (Bartee and Cheyunski, 1977). The program is being shaped by the active involvement of *problem-centered constituency groups* which help to identify management problems. The constituency groups include *resource providers* (politicians, legislators, and members of local funding agencies who control resources for local mental health centers); *technology developers* (including the center's administration, board of trustees, and support staff); *direct service providers* (e.g., psychiatrists, psychologists, social workers, and nurses); and the *service acquirers* (clients of the center as well as such indirect users as school teachers, ministers, and police department personnel). The input provided by these groups will be used in the development of learning opportunities relevant to operational settings and which can be reinforced in such settings.

The University of Alabama's Management Training Program developed by the Center for Developmental and Learning Disorders (Garove, 1975) represents an example of a multi-format approach to adult-centered learning and the reinforcement of such learning in operational settings. Designed to train management personnel for mental retardation facilities, the program consists of three basic phases: two one-week management training seminars at the university; a three-day site visit to a cooperating mental retardation facility; and eight comprehensive home-study assignments directly related to the first two phases. The primary goal of the program is to increase the managerial proficiency of each participant by linking management theory and practice. The program (described in further detail in Appendix D) places heavy emphasis on simulation exercises and on the evaluation of managerial performance.

The University of Minnesota is currently developing an independent study program for mental health administrators which will have both degree and non-degree options, and which will employ several of the methodologies mentioned above (Malban, 1975). A strategy employed by Northern Illinois University (Agranoff, 1975) is the integration of degree and non-degree students in the same courses, so that all may benefit from the others' experience and thus form a stronger link between theory and practice.

The interdisciplinary post-graduate program in mental retardation conducted by UCLA (Tarjan, 1975) over the past nine years has highlighted the important advantages of involving practitioners from various disciplines. Those with clinical backgrounds have learned more about the functions and uses of administration, while those with nonclinical backgrounds have become better informed regarding clinical practices and treatment methodologies, and their administrative implications.

These examples represent some of the innovative approaches to continuing education. The First National Conference on Education for Mental Health Administration identified additional approaches such as exchange programs for faculty members and practicing administrators, internship programs, visiting manager programs, and joint, applied research on management and organizational problems.

It is important to note that while all of these approaches hold promise, one program cannot simply copy another. The

33

particular format and learning methodologies employed will always be a function of the nature of the problem being addressed or the subject being taught, the number and types of practitioners involved, and the constraints (e.g., financial) affecting the program's setting. These factors must be assessed for each program. The following general principles and guidelines may be of some help in considering the contingencies involved:

1. The more basic and/or generic the subject matter (e.g., financial management or management theory), the greater the likelihood that a longer course (several sessions over several weeks or months) will be required to produce a useful learning experience.
2. The more specialized the subject area (e.g., management implications of legal changes, or program evaluation), the greater the likelihood that a shorter course (a two- or three-day conference or seminar) can produce a useful learning experience.
3. The greater the extent to which a course presents an overview (as opposed to in-depth coverage), the greater the likelihood that a shorter course time can produce a useful learning experience.
4. The greater the extent to which practitioners are from organizations operating in *intense environments* (Shortell, 1976), (i.e., environments characterized by high degrees of complexity, diversity, instability, uncertainty, dependence, and hostility), the greater the likelihood that a longer course will be required. Although practitioners in such environments may be under severe time constraints, various approaches such as home-study exercises, correspondence material, and telephone networks can be used to alleviate the problem.
5. The greater the extent to which practitioners are from upper management, the greater the likelihood that shorter courses may be more effective.
6. The greater the experience of the practitioners in-

volved, the greater the benefit from following an adult-centered approach.

7. The greater the diversity of the practitioner group, the greater the likelihood that longer courses will be required. This is particularly true for courses stressing interpersonal relationships and group dynamics.

8. The more unfamiliar the material is to the practitioner group, the greater the likelihood that didactic teaching methodologies (lectures and assigned readings), followed by case discussions and experiental learning, will provide a more effective learning experience.

9. The greater the extent to which learning material is conducive to graphic presentation, the greater the likelihood that television and other visual media will prove to be effective learning media.

10. The smaller the class size, the less cost effective will be the use of television and related electronic visual media.

11. The smaller the class size, the greater the likelihood that group discussions and role playing will prove to be effective learning experiences.

12. The more difficult the material, the more effective the deductive approach will usually be. The less difficult the material and the greater the extent to which it is within the realm of the practitioner's experience, the greater the effectiveness of the inductive approach. While it may appear that a deductive approach to learning is incompatible with the overall adult-centered approach which emphasizes active, experiential participation, such is not the case. Deductive and inductive approaches to learning represent ways in which knowledge is organized and communicated to others. The deductive approach does not exclude the active involvement of practitioners in its formulation and use. For example, some administrators have a highly developed philosophy of management and a conceptual map of the administrative process which should be shared with others—using a deductive ap-

proach. Thus, while it is quite easy to see the relevance of the inductive approach to adult-centered learning philosophies, one should not underestimate the continuing applicability of the deductive approach.

It also is possible to suggest some comparative advantages of specific teaching and learning methodologies, including informal lectures, cases and problem assignments, group discussions, and role playing:

Informal Lectures (planned in advance but open to student questioning and give-and-take)
1. Useful for introducing new material and for providing a background for discussion.
2. Useful for clarifying difficult material, especially through the use of examples.
3. Useful for summarizing and reviewing.

Cases and Problem Assignments
1. Useful for showing the practical application of concepts (e.g., relevance of role theory concepts for analyzing conflict in organizations).
2. Useful for increasing problem recognition and problem-solving skills.
3. Useful for reinforcing key concepts or ideas which have been discussed on a more abstract level in lectures and general class discussion.
4. Can be useful in helping the practitioner deal explicitly with different value orientations (e.g., legal changes regarding the treatment of alcoholism).

Group Discussions
1. Useful for generating new ideas, for expanding ideas and concepts and for discerning the administrative implications of new ideas and concepts (e.g., the management and planning implications of the de-institutionalization of mental health services).
2. Useful in eliciting practitioners' value orientations and for dealing with the affective component of learning.

Role Playing
1. Good for illustrating a single principle or concept which needs emphasizing.

2. Also good for developing the affective component of learning.
3. May be particularly useful in illustrating various points related to the management of conflict (e.g., conflict among members of interdisciplinary professional teams).

It is important to note that role-playing experiences should be followed up by re-integrating them into the rest of the course (e.g., by relating them to the larger issues surrounding professional teams, such as client rights and accountability to clients and funding agencies).

Some of the above propositions and suggestions have long been accepted by educators and may legitimately be termed "principles." Others are much less obvious and are subject to debate; they are best termed "assumptions" which require further testing and experimentation. They are offered as possible guidelines for those confronted with the thorny problem of how to present diverse material to heterogeneous practitioners functioning in varying sets of circumstances.

Funding

The previously mentioned survey of mental health continuing educators (Bloom, 1974) cited as a primary concern the "obtaining [of] long-term, reasonably stable general support regardless of the source of that support." It is obvious that funding needs to be obtained from multiple sources and that the primary candidates are federal funds, foundation funds, state support, tuition, and university support. Traditionally, the usual sources of "start-up and demonstration" funds have been federal and foundation grants. Some foundations, such as the Kellogg Foundation, have taken a special interest in the education of health services administrators (broadly defined) and are particularly interested in providing one or two years of "seed" money—to get a project underway while more permanent sources of funds are sought. *Such foundations should be kept informed of the importance of MH, MR/DD services and the need for improved continuing education of practicing MH, MR/DD administrators.*

However, while federal and foundation funding will remain possible sources of support, they are highly unstable sources—subject, respectively, to the vagaries of political campaigns and congressional appropriation battles, and to numerous competing interests. Thus, there is an *urgent need for stable, long-term support of continuing education efforts in the field.*

One strategy that should be pursued vigorously is the incorporation into state budgets of funds for continuing education, which would allow for ongoing staff development. It has become increasingly apparent that the efficient delivery of MH, MR/DD services is heavily dependent on the quality of available management. It would appear that persuasive arguments could be made for incorporating continuing education funds into state health and social service budgets. In blunt terms, the executive and legislative branches of state government should ask themselves, for example, why de-institutionalization of mental health patients in many states has met with so many problems (see Chapter I).

Universities (especially state universities) should also be encouraged to commit a certain percentage of funds to continuing education. Particular consideration might be given to offering stipends to individuals in difficult-to-reach, smaller, and poorly funded organizations.

It is recommended that every employing organization *establish a policy whereby administrative personnel participate in at least one continuing education activity per year.* It is further suggested that the *employing organization strive to provide at least 50 percent of the expenses associated with the continuing education* activities of its administrative personnel. A recent survey of administrators of developmental disability agencies and facilities (Drury, 1975) revealed that while the majority believed additional management training would be of benefit and that they could obtain the necessary release-time, 53 percent did not know whether their employing organization would underwrite the expense; of those that did know, 67 percent replied that their employer would *not* underwrite the expense. It will be difficult for MH, MR/DD administrators to suggest that state funds be provided for long-term support of continuing education if their employing organizations are unwilling to contribute.

Special attention should be given to meeting the continuing education needs of practitioners from states with few resources to finance such efforts. Consideration should be given to establishing regional continuing education centers to serve practitioners from surrounding states, with brief courses meeting the time and travel demands involved. Stable financial support, whether from federal, foundation, or other sources, would be essential.

Continuity and Coordination of Continuing Education Programs

Implied in the above discussion of funding stability is the need for greater continuity and coordination of continuing education. *There is need for more systematic information on the continuing education needs of practitioners, the resources available to meet these needs, and the evaluation of the various activities involved.* Consideration should be given to *establishing one continuing education coordinating center per region* which would act as a "broker" in matching demand with supply and as a catalyst in influencing the development of new programs and in the evaluation of both new and existing programs. Such coordinating centers could be based on such models as the Western Interstate Commission for Higher Education (WICHE), or the Southern Regional Educational Board (SREB). The centers would require the assistance of professional associations, state agencies, and individual delivery organizations in *establishing and enforcing criteria for continuing education, helping to develop continuing education profiles for individual administrators, and in identifying local resources.* With such structural mechanisms, it would be possible to develop a more systematic continuing education effort, rather than the episodic approaches characteristic of much of the current training.

We suggest that the above recommendations be carefully considered and analyzed. A reasonable strategy would be to establish coordinating centers in one or two regions to test their viability and to determine the types of problems encountered. After a few years' experience, it might be possible to extend the concept to other regions.

V

Quality Assessment
and Licensure and Certification Issues

As mental health and mental retardation/developmental disabilities (MH, MR/DD) continuing education develops, the issues of program accreditation and individual assessment and recognition will assume increasing importance. These issues are, of course, interrelated since criteria for individual assessment and recognition are frequently based on the quality of the continuing education experience as determined by accreditation and related mechanisms. The following sections briefly summarize some of the issues involved and offer several suggestions.

Quality of Assessment of Continuing
Education Programs

Although not without drawbacks, *accreditation of educational programs* by outside groups is a powerful mechanism for, at least, assuring minimum standards of quality. The increasing proliferation of accrediting agencies is a major problem in the health manpower field (Roemer, 1973). Therefore, careful consideration should be given to the various alternatives for accrediting MH, MR/DD continuing education programs. The development of accreditation criteria by various professional groups represents one alternative. A second alternative is the formation of a multi-disciplinary accrediting body composed of members from MH, MR/DD administration and related fields. *A third alternative is to build on existing bodies which accredit the various professional schools in which continuing education programs are conducted*—for example, the Accrediting Commission on Graduate Education for Health Services Administration and the accrediting bodies for schools of business administration, public administration/public affairs, and psychiatry. While the latter approach suffers in that the various professional schools have different accreditation requirements, it might be possible for their accrediting groups to agree on a basic set of criteria for reviewing MH, MR/DD continuing education programs in their respective schools. These accrediting bodies should be encouraged to review the non–university-based programs as well. Health-related professional associations could also play an important role by helping current accrediting bodies develop relevant criteria and by providing the necessary technical assistance. This strategy seems preferable to adding more groups to an already fragmented accreditation system.

Regardless of the particular mechanism which might be established, the following are offered as examples of criteria which should be considered for nationwide application. While primarily directed at university-based or affiliated programs, all items except 1, 3, and 5 are applicable to non–university-based efforts as well.

1. Primary responsibility for the program must reside within an established department or school of the university.
2. Primary responsibility for the program must be delegated to a specific individual (or group).
3. At least 50 percent of the continuing education faculty must be drawn from the full-time faculty of the university.

4. Faculty quality must be evidenced by either a doctoral degree in a relevant field or an equivalent combination of relevant graduate work and teaching or work experience.
5. With regard to criteria for promotion and advancement, teaching in the continuing education program must be accorded equal weight with other teaching responsibilities.
6. The program should have a clear statement of objectives which is reflected in the activities and content of the program.
7. The program must show evidence of established working relationships with local delivery settings and practitioners.
8. The program must show evidence of viable financial support, including that of the parent department or school.
9. The program must provide library resources appropriate for the continuing education of MH, MR/DD administrators, i.e., the specialized materials relevant to the administration of MH, MR/DD services.
10. There must be an established plan for the evaluation of course offerings and program content.
11. Faculty must show evidence of active involvement in research relevant to the further development of MH, MR/DD administration.

No specific criteria for curriculum content are offered, since the content will vary according to the needs of participating practitioners. It would be expected, however, that the curriculum would include much of the content outlined in Chapter III. In brief, the criteria are directed at the outputs and the inputs and inflows (in the belief that a certain minimum level of inputs and inflows is necessary for a quality program). No criteria are provided for the transformation process, since the individuals involved, both faculty and practitioners, should be left free to experiment and innovate.

Individual Assessment and Recognition

The following recommendations and suggestions are made regarding individual assessment and recognition:

1. *Priority should be given to the granting of academic credit.* This is consistent with the concept of rigorous, analytically oriented courses, primarily university-based or affiliated, taught by faculty of the same caliber available to full-time graduate students. Some universities have developed the *continuing education unit* (CEU) concept in which a predetermined number of academic credits is granted for a given number of continuing education courses.

2. *Certification* is an appropriate form of recognition when an individual has completed a number of basic courses toward a master's degree or has completed a number of courses in a specialty area such as financial management or operations research.

3. Given the increasing demand for public accountability and given the experience with licensure in the nursing home field, it is possible that in the future licensure may be required for MH, MR/DD administrators. In this event, the following recommendations are suggested for consideration:

    a) That minimal sets of standards for licensure be established on a *nationwide* basis.

    b) That a combination of formal administrative academic training and work experience be required for licensure with *relevant work experience substituting for lack of a master's degree in an administrative field* (for example, health services administration, public administration, business administration). For those without an appropriate master's degree, a scheme relating years of administrative work experience to the appropriate level of responsibility should be worked out; for example, at least two years for middle managers and at least three years for chief administrative officers. It is further suggested that *those with an appropriate master's degree be required to have at least one year of work experience before licensure.*

c) That all individuals, regardless of previous background, *have successfully completed at least one continuing education course during the two years* before licensure or certification.

d) That the individual *successfully pass a standardized national examination which would test his knowledge and skills in MH, MR/DD administration.* It is suggested that this examination have a common section devoted to basic principles of managerial practice, organization behavior, and financial management and special sections devoted to particular problems of MH, MR/DD administration. It might be suggested that an individual, in addition to choosing the special section related to his or her own field, be required to complete at least one of the other two subsections. This may encourage the individual to learn more about a different but highly related field, thus fostering the development of "integrative" thinking demanded by the field of MH, MR/DD administration.

4. If a licensing board is formed, it is important that it be made up of representatives from professional groups such as the Association of Mental Health Administrators, the American Psychiatric Association, and the Association of University Affiliated Programs; from the academic community; and from the public.

5. It is recommended that the *initial period of licensure be five years.* At the end of the first five years, it is recommended that re-licensure be based either on the successful completion of the equivalent of at least six continuing education units or on satisfactory completion of proficiency in at least two areas of MH, MR/DD administration. It is recommended that, *at the end*

of ten years, relicensure be based on *both* successful completion of the national examination and six
additional continuing education units.

6. An alternative to licensure is certification by a relevant professional group. Again, the various professional groups representing the fields of MH, MR/DD
administration *might find it advantageous to develop
common core criteria*—to be supplemented by specialized criteria which might vary from one field to
another. The remainder of the recommendations for
licensure would apply also to certification.

In making the above recommendations, emphasis has been
placed on maintaining a balance between assuring competence and providing mobility. Requiring written examinations
and continuing education course work for licensure or certification is designed to ensure at least minimal levels of competence. Applying criteria on a nationwide basis helps to assure geographic mobility.

Whatever groups become involved in accreditation, licensure, and certification, *it is important that coordination be
established among the regional continuing education coordinating centers and the state agencies* mentioned in Chapter
IV. If funding at the state level is to be based in part on
certification or licensure of MH, MR/DD administrators,
then the state agencies must be kept informed regarding the
standards involved and the status of particular individuals at
particular times. The regional coordinating centers for continuing education must also be kept informed, in order to ensure
that the process of matching participant needs and interests
with course offerings is also relevant to licensure and/or certification requirements.

VI

Summary of Recommendations:
Bringing the Target into Sharper Focus

This monograph began by describing the complexities faced by administrators of mental health and mental retardation/developmental disabilities (MH, MR/DD) services. Thompson's definition of administration as "shooting at a moving target" was cited as emphasizing the complexities of the managerial role in terms of the technical, political, and visionary skills required for effective performance. A working definition of continuing education was presented, together with an open systems framework for conceptualizing the continuing education process and for developing continuing education programs. This was followed by an assessment of particular needs of MH, MR/DD administration, the presentation of several matrix approaches to curriculum content, and a discussion of the importance of evaluation. Relevant implementation strategies and appropriate learning methodologies were then discussed, followed by an examination of accreditation, licensure, and certification issues. The major recommendations and emphases of the report are summarized below.

Chapter I

1. Distinctive characteristics of MH, MR/DD administration, as compared to other forms of health services
administration, include: (1) a somewhat more extended network of external environmental relationships which must be maintained, particularly in regard
to consumer involvement; (2) the difficulties involved
in measuring outcomes; and (3) the stigma associated
with many of the conditions presented by clients.
MH, MR/DD continuing education programs must
reflect the managerial implications of these differences.

2. The similarities between mental health and mental
retardation/developmental disabilities administration
are sufficient for a monograph on continuing education
to be addressed to both groups. Further, appropriately designed continuing education programs can
serve both groups.

3. Managerial skills in the delivery of MH, MR/DD
services are in great demand. Since only a small part
of the present and near-future demand will be met
by new graduates, there is need for the development
of high quality continuing education programs for
existing practitioners.

Chapter II

4. Because of the contingencies involved (practitioner
background, type of organization, size of organization,
etc.) in the continuing education process and the
experience which practitioners bring to the learning
environment, greater emphasis should be placed on
learning models based on the *mutual participation of
faculty and practitioners.*

5. Continuing education efforts must be *continually
evaluated* in regard to the motivation of the applicant
to the program, the quality of program faculty and

curriculum, and the nature of the changes (if any) which take place as the result of the program.

6. There is *no single best organizational location* for conducting continuing education. Those programs which happen to be based in or associated with universities should *capitalize on the strengths* of particular universities, departments, and schools, and this will vary from campus to campus.

7. Continuing education is defined as the *planned learning*, beyond the basic professional education, of *generic* administrative skills relevant to the delivery of MH, MR/DD services. The emphasis is on specific learning objectives geared to the development of additional managerial knowledge, skill, and value insights which will be useful to the administrator in a number of different situations.

8. The advantage of an *open systems* approach to continuing education is that it emphasizes the *interdependence* and *dynamics* of continuing education activities as well as the principles of *equifinality* (different ways of reaching the same goal) and *multifinality* (similar initial conditions leading to possibly dissimilar end states).

Chapter III

9. *Careful assessments must be made of practitioner needs*, taking into account such variables as practitioner background, type of employing organization, stage of career, and the manager's position within the organization. Items for consideration would include training in basic management and organization theory, planning, accounting and financial management, small-group dynamics and interpersonal skills, and community politics and inter-organizational decision making.

10. *Matrix approaches* to relating practitioner needs to academic disciplines and knowledge areas are useful

in obtaining overviews of the resources and alternatives available for designing particular programs. Matrices may be constructed at varying levels of concreteness in regard to both practitioner needs and academic disciplines and knowledge areas.

11. Greater attention should be given to *impact evaluations* of continuing education programs.

Chapter IV

12. While continuing education programs may be conducted in a variety of settings (see point 6 above), they must be focused on *the needs of MH, MR/DD administrators*, and *there must be involvement with local delivery sites* where these are available.

13. MH, MR/DD continuing education efforts which exist on the same campus or in the same geographic area should be coordinated to avoid duplication of effort.

14. The faculty involved in the continuing education effort should be *of the same quality* as that available to full-time graduate students.

15. In evaluating faculty performance, the teaching of continuing education courses *should receive the same recognition* as the teaching of full-time graduate students.

16. Where qualified practitioners are available, they should be actively involved in the teaching process. If appropriate, the joint development of courses by a faculty member and a practitioner should be encouraged.

17. As implied in point 4 above, greater attention needs to be given to "adult-centered" approaches to learning. This includes considering the need for *reinforcing* formal education with direct, on-the-job application.

18. There is an urgent need for *stable, long-term support* of MH, MR/DD continuing education. Serious con-

sideration should be given to *incorporating* funds for continuing education in *federal, state, agency, and university budgets.*

19. Every MH, MR/DD delivery organization should be encouraged to establish a policy requiring administrative personnel to participate in *at least one continuing education activity per year.* The employing organization should be encouraged to *develop budget and financing mechanisms to meet at least 50 percent* of the tuition and travel expenses.

20. There is a great need for *more systematic information* on the continuing education needs of practitioners, the resources available to meet these needs, and evaluations of the efforts involved. Toward this end, it is suggested that *continuing education coordinating centers* be initiated on a demonstration basis in one or two regions. If judged useful, they might be extended throughout the country. These centers would act as "brokers" in helping to match demand with supply and would work closely with professional associations, state agencies, and individual delivery organizations in developing individual and organizational continuing education profiles, in identifying resources, and in clarifying criteria.

Chapter V

21. While many approaches are available for accrediting MH, MR/DD continuing education, serious consideration should be given to *building upon existing accrediting agencies* rather than to creating new agencies which would further fragment the accreditation process.

22. To promote at least a minimal level of quality, accreditation should be *based on nationwide standards.*

23. In regard to participant recognition, *first priority should be given to the granting of academic credit.*

24. *Certification* is also an appropriate form of recogni-

tion in cases where the individual has completed a certain number of courses, *particularly in specialty areas* (for example, financial management).

25. *In the event of nationwide licensure and/or certification requirements*, the following are recommended:

    a) *Relevant work experience should be accepted as partial substitution for academic coursework.*

    b) All individuals should be required to *complete successfully at least one continuing education course* during the two years before licensure or certification.

    c) All individuals *shall be required to pass a national standardized examination* testing the administrator's knowledge of administrative theory and practice as applied to MH, MR/DD administration.

    d) *The initial licensure should be for a period of five years*, at the end of which re-licensure should require *successful completion of at least six academic credit hours of continuing education, or demonstration of proficiency (through testing) of at least two areas of MH, MR/DD administration.*

    e) *At the end of ten years*, re-licensure or re-certification should require *both* successful completion of at least six academic credit hours of continuing education and successful completion of a national examination testing proficiency in various areas of MH, MR/DD administration.

26. Whatever groups may become involved in accreditation, licensure, and certification activities, it is important that *close coordinating ties be established* with state agencies and the regional continuing education coordinating centers.

The above recommendations take on added significance when considered in the light of urgent needs for improved

52

administration of MH, MR/DD services. For example, a recent United States General Accounting Office evaluation of the management of community mental health centers stressed the need for improved performance in *needs assessment and planning for delivery, mechanisms of consumer participation, management practices, and in the development of coordinated systems of services* (United States General Accounting Office, 1974). Examples of the negative effect of poor administration on delivery of services include the earlier-cited example involving de-institutionalization of services, the lack of coordinated admission policies for state hospitals, programs funded out of proportion to stated goals, the inability to develop goals and priorities, and deficiencies in gathering and analyzing data for program implementation and evaluation. In addition, MH, MR/DD administrators are facing a series of new issues, including changing societal expectations regarding mental health, the impact of new technology, and the effect of new sources of funding. (See Appendix E for issues identified by the Western Interstate Commission on Higher Education.)

Finally, it should be noted that these recommendations and the general thrust of this report reinforce those of the report of the Commission on Education for Health Administration (*Education for Health Administration*, 1975). Among the general recommendations of that report were:

Responding to unmet educational needs. Additional demands for education must be anticipated. Practitioners who have not had previous health administration education, or who were educated in the past and now need updated knowledge, attitudes, and skills, as well as those wishing to enter practice, will seek educational opportunities.

Developing lifelong learning opportunities. Promoting and providing for the continuing competence of practicing health administrators, whether or not they have had formal health administration education, is seen as one of the most important issues facing health administration education today.

References

Agranoff, R., Coordinator, Mental Health Administrative Program, Northern Illinois University, Personal Communication, 1975.

Argyris, C. and D. A. Schon, *Theory in Practice: Increasing Professional Effectiveness* (San Francisco: Jossey-Bass Publishers, 1974).

Bartee, E. M. and F. Cheyunski, "A Methodology for Process-Oriented Organizational Diagnosis," *The Journal of Applied Behavioral Science* 13, no. 1 (1977).

Becker, G., *Human Capital* (New York: Columbia University Press, 1964).

Becker, S. and D. Neuhauser, *The Efficient Organization* (New York: Elsevier, 1975).

Blake, R. and J. Mouton, *The Managerial Grid* (Houston: Gulf Publishing Co., 1964).

Bloom, B., "Current Issues in Mental Health Continuing Education," *Mental Health Continuing Education in the West* 1 (Fall, 1974) 16.

Boissoneau, R., "The Continuing Education Role of Graduate Studies in Health Services Management," University of Missouri, Columbia, 1975.

Cahill, P., *Final Report of the First National Conference on Education for Mental Health Administration* (Washington, D.C.: Association of University Programs in Health Administration, June, 1975).

Campbell, D. T. and J. C. Stanley, *Experimental and Quasi-Experimental Designs for Research* (Chicago: Rand McNally, 1966).

Caplan, G., "Announcing a Continuing Education Program for Mental Health Planners-Administrators," Harvard Medical School, Laboratory of Community Psychiatry, 1974.

Committee on Standards, *Guidelines and Standards for Professional Master's Degree Programs in Public Affairs, Public Administration* (Washington, D.C.: National Association of Schools of Public Affairs and Administration, 1975).

"Costs of Evaluation," Proceedings: *Evaluation in Continuing Medical Education*, Kansas City, Kansas, University of Kansas Medical Center, August 30, 1970, p. 28.

Dolgoff, T., "Continuing Education for Mental Health Administrators," Menninger Foundation, Topeka, Kansas, 1975.

Drury, J. D., "A Management and Interest Study of Administrators of Agencies and Facilities for the Developmentally Disabled," University of Missouri, Columbia, 1975.

Education for Health Administration, Volume 1, (Ann Arbor: Health Administration Press, 1975).

Elder, J. et al., *Education of Health Services Administrators in an Interdisciplinary Model*, Revised Edition, University of Oregon Health Services Center, January, 1976.

Feldman, S., *The Administration of Mental Health Services* (Springfield, Illinois: Charles C. Thomas, 1973).

Foley, A., "Perspectives in Continuing Education," Paper Presented at the First National Conference on Education for Mental Health Administration, New Orleans, Louisiana, March 5-7, 1975.

Garove, W., "Overview: Management Training Program," Center for Developmental and Learning Disorders, University of Alabama in Birmingham, 1975.

Katz, D. and R. L. Kahn, *The Social Psychology of Organizations* (New York: John Wiley and Sons, 1966).

Knowles, M., "Human Resources Development in OD," *Public Administration Review* 34 (March/April, 1974): 116.

Lawrence, P. and J. Lorsch, *Organization and Environment* (Cambridge: Harvard University Press, 1967).

Malban, J., *Independent Study Program for Mental Health Administrators*, working draft, University of Minnesota, June, 1975.

"Mental Health Administration Continuing Education Program," Tulane University, School of Public Health and Tropical Medicine, 1975.

"Perspectives on Mental Health and Mental Retardation Administration," *Program Notes, Association of University Programs in Health Administration*, 63 (February, 1975).

Roemer, R., "Social Regulation of Health Manpower," in *Fostering the Growing Need to Learn*, Division of Regional Medical Programs, Health Resources Administration, Rockville, Maryland, July, 1973, pp. 369–410.

Schultz, T. ed., "Investment in Human Beings," *Journal of Political Economy* 70 (October, 1962), Part 2.

Shortell, S. M., "The Role of Environment in a Configurational Theory of Organizations," *Human Relations* (in press, 1976).

Shortell, S. M. and W. C. Richardson, *Health Program Evaluation* (St. Louis: C. V. Mosby and Co., forthcoming, 1978).

Tarjan, G., Personal Interview (1975).

Thompson, J. D., *Organizations in Action* (New York: McGraw-Hill, 1967).

U. S. General Accounting Office, *Need for More Effective Management of Community Mental Health Centers Program*, B-164031 (5), Comptroller General's Report to the Congress (Washington, D.C.: GAD, 1974), pp. 1–69.

Von Bertalanffy, L., *General Systems Theory: Foundations, Development, Applications* (New York: G. Braziller, 1968).

Yolles, S., "The Importance of Administration in Mental Health," Paper Presented at the First National Conference on Education for Mental Health Administration, New Orleans, Louisiana, March 5-7, 1975.

APPENDIX A

A Methodology for Process-Oriented Organizational Diagnosis

Edwin M. Bartee and Fred Cheyunski
Vanderbilt University

Possibly one of the most important issues in organizational and community change is the manner in which an intervention can facilitate change processes.[1] The first step in such an intervention is diagnostic. The purpose of such a diagnosis is to produce a new level of awareness within the system, which in turn will result in cultural and structural changes (Dalton, 1970; Lorsch and Lawrence, 1972).

Traditional Awareness-Raising (Diagnostic) Techniques

Several diagnostic techniques are suggested in the literature as useful approaches in facilitating awareness-raising processes. One of these is the *survey research* technique (Likert, 1967; Taylor and Bowers, 1972). In this approach the interventionist develops an instrument that contains a set of questions designed to collect specific information considered by the former as important in the anticipated change program. The questions usually ask about attitudes toward supervisors, peers, and subordinates; knowledge of communication systems; perception of organizational relationships; and so on. Survey research questionnaires reflect certain explicit and implicit judgments about what is valued in an organization by the designer of the instrument. For example, an overriding value that could be communicated by a questionnaire is that collaborative rather than authoritarian styles of management enhance organizational morale and production.

A second technique for diagnosis is the *interview* (Gorden, 1969; Matarazzo and Wiens, 1972). In this approach, a third party engages in a personal dialogue with members of the client system and obtains information similar in character to that collected in survey research. The interview has the potential of acquiring more in-depth information with greater

[1] This paper represents the first of a series of research reports that will evolve from the activities of the Center for Research on Human Service Systems, Vanderbilt University. Funding support is provided by NIMH, NIH, and the State of Tennessee.

clarity and a sense of the feelings of the person interviewed in relation to a particular issue. The potential for data to be influenced by the value judgments of the interviewer is also greater. In our opinion the "objectivity" of the predesigned questionnaire is lost and the chances for the verbal statements of an interviewee to be overtly or covertly biased by the interviewer are obvious.

A third technique for diagnosis is *participant observation* (Heyns and Lippitt, 1954; Klein, 1966), which provides information qualitatively different from the other two techniques. In this case, a third party makes trained observations on the behavior and interactions of clients as they function in their "natural habitats." It is therefore possible to observe, record, and interpret the *behavior* of the client with this technique, but the potential for the value bias of the observer to influence the resulting information is probably greater than with either of the previously mentioned techniques—even if more than one observer, precoded behavior check lists, and/or videotapes are used.[2]

In other words, the information collected by questionnaire or interview method at least represents an introduction of perceptions of both the client and the data collector. The present "awareness" of the interviewee is recorded.

There are diagnostic interventions that use a combination of these techniques (Levinson, 1972). The information derived from one or more of these techniques is compiled by the third party, interpreted, and "fed back" to the client system. This is usually done by distributing written output data followed by diagnosis feedback discussion sessions conducted in some small-group format (Alderfer and Brown, 1972; Miles et al., 1969; Neff, 1965).

Client participation in this process is usually limited to the rather passive roles of giving information to and receiving information from a third party. The data to be collected are determined by this third party, whether through questionnaire

---

[2] A variation of this technique would be the use of audio-taping of conversations from which implications would be deduced by a third party (Argyris, 1970).

construction, formulation of interview questions, or notation of observed behavior. The categories imposed in the data gathering and in the feedback process amount to a manipulation of the client's information content. Client data generation is restricted, and client responsibility for the data and their subsequent use tends to be given over to the third party, thereby diminishing the possibility of client-initiated action. The likelihood of effective intervention is less probable because of incomplete information and limited client ownership of the data and any subsequent action plan. We call these approaches content-influential to underscore a process in which the role of the client is one of passive information giving and receiving; the information content is collected, analyzed, interpreted, fed back (and consequently biased) by the third party.

Self-Diagnosis: Process versus Content

The methodology set forth below is designed to reduce the number of ineffective interventions by providing a means to direct attention away from the personality and style of the third party (who may be ineffective due to his or her own personal limitations or to problems inherent in the system), and to focus attention on the perceptions of problems of the client system.

In the approach that will be described, the clients are viewed not only as the *individuals* who bring in and pay the consultant but also as *groups* which are formed to represent the constituencies of the organization. Those individuals in the client system who bring the consultant in are typically persons who are looking for ways in which their organization can become more effective in dealing with its problems. Those persons are usually referred to the consultant by someone known to them, and they have a willingness to try the approach proposed. Their commitment most often is to the diagnostic process as an initial stage of a change effort. Part of the procedure, which will be elaborated below, includes the defining and assembling of constituency groups from among the members of the client system. Once these groups have been formed, the task of the consultant becomes one of working with these groups as his/her "clients," as well as with the key individuals.

During the critical entry period, this method provides a *structure* which allows the consultant to be quite authoritative, but at the same time minimizes the interference with the *content* of the clients' information. In fact, it is important for the interventionist to control the *process* to enable the clients to generate and control their own information and awareness. The consultant uses the methodology to establish and reinforce norms of group interaction and to establish a relationship in which the clients can become more and more independent. This leadership style, which is transferable to the clients, allows the interventionist to create a situation in which his/her personal skills can be most useful and can assist the clients to do the same.

We are suggesting here that the potential for ultimate change within an organization may be enhanced by the use of diagnostic techniques that are more *process oriented.* We hypothesize that *self-diagnosis* by the members of an organization should increase the potential for long-range change because (1) it will tend to create cognitive dissonance (Festinger, 1957) in relation to the clients' own internal situation and minimize the dissonance between the interventionist and the client; and (2) it should tend to facilitate the development of change mechanisms internal to the organization by allowing a greater initial ownership of its change program. The chances for obtaining these basic goals will be greater if the particular diagnosis and feedback method used incorporates the following characteristics, which are process oriented:

1. The client system becomes the authority in determining what information is important to share.
2. The clients immediately tend to own and take responsibility for the data generated.
3. The interventionist facilitates only the process by

which the data are generated and shared. The data which are produced by the clients are communicated in the terms that are best understood by the clients. The format in which the data are to be shared should maximize the potential for taking effective action in response to the data.

4. The process by which the data are produced will tend to maximize probability that the clients will take effective action.

A Methodology for Process-Oriented Diagnosis

This methodology is based upon the assumption that organizational dynamics consist of complex interactions, e.g., recognition of power relationships, differentiation of roles and decision-making responsibilities and so on between four primary constituencies that represent significantly different, but equally valid, viewpoints of an organization and its problems. Organizational members have different cognitive structures that they use for understanding their positions or roles in the organization (Zajonc and Wolfe, 1966). It is suggested here that the taxonomy of these different cognitive structures can be described in terms of the following constituencies:

1. *Resource-providers* include those groups and individuals who require, and provide resources such as money, information, and other forms of legitimization from the environment. For a business firm this constituency would include members of the board of directors, trade associations, banks, government control agencies, and others. A social-service agency would include members of the board of directors, government funding agencies, banks, etc., in its resource-providers constituency.

2. *Technology-developers* include the groups and individuals that manage and administer the organization so that the resources are converted in a way that the technologies of the organization will be developed.

65

The technologies for a business firm may produce either products or services. The technology-developers are those managers and administrators who determine the policies and procedures for utilizing resources in the production of the products or services. In the case of the social-service agency the members of this constituency would be the agency director and the administrative staff that determines the application of resources for delivering the particular social service.

3. *Direct-service providers* include those groups and individuals who consistently interact directly with the customers or clientele of the organization in the sale or delivery of its product or service. For a business firm the members of this constituency would be those persons who function in direct relationship with the customer: sales, marketing, quality control, delivery. In the social-service agency these persons may be doctors, professional counselors, therapists, social workers, depending upon the particular nature of the social service that is delivered.

4. *Service-acquirers* include the customers or clientele of an organization. Wholesalers, distributors, retailers, and consumers represent the service-acquirers constituency for the business firm. For the social-service agency the general public that serves as clientele to the agency represents this constituency.

These four basic constituencies exist for any organizational unit whether it be a department, branch, or total organization. The first step in the methodology is the *determination of the organizational unit* that is to be the object for diagnosis by those who are employing the consultant, with his/her guidance. If it is a department of a larger organization, the four constituencies would be different from those of a total organization.

For example, suppose that the organizational unit were defined as a particular school in a city system: a high school. In identifying the constituencies for this situation, (1) the resource-providers would include the local governing body in the city, the board of education, and other units of the school system that provide or make determinations in relation to the provision of resources such as money, supplies, equipment, facilities, etc.; (2) the technology-developers would include the school principal and other administrators within the school; (3) the direct-service providers would include the teachers and others who make regular direct contact with the students for the purpose of providing education and instruction; and (4) the service-acquirers would be the students, their parents, and the community served.

Constituency Groups

A group of people selected to represent one or more of the four constituencies is called a *constituency group*. Once the organizational unit is determined, the next step is for the consultant and the individuals within the organization that are retaining his/her services to *design the constituency group or groups*. This task can be and, in the authors' experience, has been done by groups brought together by a chairman of the board or a top-management person within the organization to work with the consultants in planning this aspect of the intervention. If the organizational unit is quite small there may be no justification for more than one group. When this is the case it is desirable to constitute the group so that the four constituencies are represented by equal numbers of people. The ideal size for a group is eight people (although a group may range in size from six to ten people), and if only one group is formed it could consist of two people from each of the constituencies.

There are two primary criteria for selecting individuals for a constituency group.

1. The persons must have roles which properly fit within the particular constituency.
2. The individuals must have been sufficiently involved in the activities of the constituency to ensure that they

possess a significant amount of information of potential value to the organization.

The candidates may have several roles in the organizational unit. The critical factor that should determine their qualification as constituency-group members is the degree of *relevant information* that the persons have in the particular roles they hold; this determination is usually best made by those retaining the consultant in conjunction with others that have been involved in planning the workshop. The primary purpose of the diagnosis is to identify and understand the important problems that exist in relation to the organizational unit as perceived by each constituency. To do this successfully it is important that the groups representing each constituency contain members who function regularly over time in a role of that constituency. When these conditions are met, it is assumed that these persons will serve as important information sources.

The size of the constituency groups is important. The trade-off here is to design the group large enough so that a "group culture" can exist but, at the same time, not have the group so large that there is not sufficient opportunity for individual participation. If the size of the organizational unit is large, an optimal number of groups would be four, one for each constituency. It is thus assumed that each of the constituency groups would be a "representative sample" of its total constituency and thereby reflect a unique bias of that constituency in the organizational diagnosis process. Encouraging all members to share a sense of active participation in the process might be accomplished by making the formation of the groups a political process, i.e., *election* of persons to represent a constituency. It is further assumed that a comprehensive organizational diagnosis is only possible when the problem biases of all four constituencies are included. The process *can* be conducted with less than all four constituencies included, but this would yield incomplete information and would constitute only a partial diagnosis, of questionable benefit to the system or overall client.

Stratified constituency groups. When a particular constituency is quite large (as the service-acquirers generally are), it may prove desirable to form more than one constituency group (i.e., stratified constituency groups) to enhance the likelihood that the primary characteristics of the population will be adequately represented. An important degree of stratification may be found in the constituency population that needs to be considered when the groups are designed. For example, in the high school case mentioned above, the service-acquirers would have an important stratification between students and parents. It could prove desirable to form separate groups of students and parents, both of which would represent the service-acquirers constituency for the high school.

The Problem Diagnosis Workshop

The initial diagnosis and the initial intervention for the organizational unit is achieved as the consultant conducts a *problem diagnosis workshop.* The ideal workshop includes all four constituency groups, although it can be conducted with as few as one. There is a "social advantage" to having all of the constituencies experience one another even though they remain separate as groups during the process of the workshop. The organizational unit tends to take on a new dimension for the participants as they become aware of the four constituencies in action.[3]

The general process of the workshop is as follows:

1. Each group identifies a *general problem area.* This may be done as a predetermined area of concern, or each group may be asked to determine an area collaboratively.
2. For the general problem area, each group identifies and describes the *present situation* according to a structured procedure (described below).

[3] Subsequent experience in using this model has indicated that the social advantage may be nullified by the level of threat that is generated by all four groups' meeting together. This issue will be dealt with in more detail in later reports.

3. After gaining a sense of the present situation, each group collaborates in producing a list of ideal *desired situations* using the same structured procedure.
4. Each group determines its *priority-desired situation*.
5. The problem is then defined in the following manner: *the problem is to change the present situation so that it becomes the priority-desired situation* (Bartee, 1973).

Each group goes through this process independently of the other groups under the process direction of the consultant and other group facilitators who are trained in using the method. The facilitator's role is to lead the group through a structured process that is designed to enhance the quantity and quality of information that is obtained from the group. The process gives emphasis to both the individual and group modes of generating information. In this methodology, the individual is treated as the basic element of organizational life, and the process is designed to provide the opportunity for individuals in a management situation to influence their immediate environment in a way that maximizes their perceived self-interest. Individuals are allowed to decide for themselves what information to share within the group as well as what risks they will take in order to influence their situation. An atmosphere that allows for personal sharing and encourages group confidentiality is thus fostered.

The workshop is designed to obtain particular conceptual data from individuals who have information relating to one or more of the basic constituencies. This particular process is enhanced when the individuals have an opportunity to be introspective and reflective in relation to the general problem area. It is critically important that the ideas of which the individual becomes aware are recorded. The *process of recording* "releases" the data from the individual's short-term memory so that another idea may be recalled from long-term memory and brought into immediate consciousness (Simon and Newell, 1970). The written items also serve as external artifacts that will provide a stimulus to the recall of more data in relation to each specific item.

The workshop is also oriented to stimulate *collaboration among individuals* in a group to produce information. To accomplish this goal the group facilitator leads the group in the following process (Delbecq and Van de Ven, 1971):*

1. Each individual *writes* short statements that describe the person's perception of the focus of attention in a particular session.
2. Each group member verbally shares, in turn, an item on his written list with the other group members.
3. Each shared item is written on a display sheet so that all members of the group can read it.
4. As each item is shared in turn by a group member, the other members make certain that they *understand what the person intends* by the particular statement. The emphasis is on understanding and clarification and not on evaluation, agreement, or disagreement.
5. For each shared item the other members of the group are given an opportunity to indicate whether they have an item on their list that corresponds to or is identical to the shared item. This determination should be made by all persons in relation to their statements. If the person judges that a particular shared statement does not satisfactorily include his, the opportunity to include it in the group list will be provided later.
6. The above process ends when each group member is satisfied that all his or her information is accurately represented on the group list, either as a specific item on the list or included in the items submitted by others. The effect of this process is to balance the degree of

* The authors have been strongly influenced by the work of André Delbecq in the development of this methodology, particularly in the use of the nominal group technique. The authors have made modifications to Delbecq's approach, which generally reflect the fact that the technique was originally developed for application to a community program planning situation, whereas the present application is intended for intraorganizational diagnosis. Though the authors are indebted to Delbecq for this very positive influence, at the same time they assume full responsibility for their own interpretations and modifications of this pioneering work.

influence that each person has and to encourage openness. (When influence is felt to be unbalanced, it tends to inhibit the sharing of information.)

7. After such information is recorded, the group is provided an opportunity to discuss, evaluate, support, and criticize the various data.

8. After the discussion is complete, if the group is to set priorities among the items on the list, each member should be allowed to vote for the items that he considers to be most important. Once these votes are tallied, a further discussion by the group should be conducted in order to reach a satisfactory *group consensus*, indicated by an emphasis on one or more of the priority items or by some statement combining several items. This step is often "much easier said than done." Quite often the facilitator has to take an active role in questioning and probing the group and its individual members to assist in their arriving at a consensus.

The above procedure is followed for *each of the steps* described previously. The combined methodology for the problem diagnosis workshop follows:

1. The *general problem area* is discussed and understood by the members of the group. Discussion should be limited to information giving, receiving, and clarification. Any attempts by the group to engage in problem solving (i.e., speculation on possible solutions, preoccupation with the possibility of solution, or expressed concerns for implementation) should be discouraged by the facilitator.

2. Once the general problem area is clearly stated and understood by the group, all members, working alone as individuals but in the presence of others in the group, are asked to list on a sheet of paper all of the descriptive statements that they can think of which describe the *present situation* as it relates to the general problem area. Each person should be allowed to

take all of the time he or she needs in this listing process.

3.   Once each individual has completed the description of the present situation, the group is then asked to collaborate in exchanging the information. This is accomplished by the individuals', in turn, sharing one of their statements that describes the present situation. After the person's statement is written up before the group to the satisfaction of the individual, the other members of the group are provided with opportunity to obtain clarification. Attempts by other group members to evaluate or compare the person's statement in any way are discouraged. Once clarification is obtained the other group members are asked to indicate whether they have an item on their lists similar to the item just posted. If so, they indicate this corresponding item, and a tally of agreements is kept on the display sheet. This procedure is continued until all items on the individual lists have been included to the satisfaction of each group member.

4.   The group members are then asked to freely discuss the *group perception* of the present situation with one another. This should be an unrestricted discussion that allows evaluation, opinion-giving, or whatever. Although the group facilitator remains with the group, during this period his or her comments are limited to process observations.

5.   Once there is general agreement that all aspects of the present situation have been satisfactorily described, group members are asked, as before, to work alone as individuals but in the presence of others in the group. They are now asked to list all of the statements pertaining to aspects of the present situation with which they are dissatisfied and write alongside each, a statement that describes the person's fantasy of a *desired situation*. Persons are encouraged to be as idealistic as possible in making their statements without any concern for practicality. When all group

members have completed their lists, the information is exchanged and discussed in the same way as in (3) and (4) above.

6. In contrast to the process steps to define the present situation, the desired situation items are assigned priorities. As stated previously, it is suggested that a "straw vote" be used to facilitate this process. The final tallies are not intended to restrict the group's later action, but to provide an opportunity for focusing further discussion and priority decisions. Experience has shown that a good indication of consensus can be obtained by asking each member of the group to vote for five of the items posted and to have these votes tallied.

7. The structured methodology is complete when a set of *problem definitions* is produced by each group. The number of problem definitions is determined by the number of priority-desired situations that have been agreed on. A problem is identified as what *has to be changed in the present situation to achieve the priority-desired situation.* Since the "problem" constitutes the difference between the present situation and the desired situation, it suggests some action or change that would be necessary but does not define the specific changes nor advocate the action. The workshop ends with the listing of these priority problems by each group and the completion of any discussion that follows.

Comments On Group Process and Workshop Design

The basic purpose in facilitating a constituency group in this workshop is to help create conditions within the group that will encourage its members to share information. Persons in general tend to "sit on" information in a situation that is experienced as threatening in any way. Such feelings of threat are reinforced by the tendency for members of a group to evaluate a person's contribution rather than to accept the information as valid for the person who is pro-

74

viding it. The tendency in such cases is for a group to provide the information that is held by those with the most skill and experience in dominating and controlling a group situation. Though the information from these persons is important, the information from all group members is of potentially equal importance in a constituency or nominal group design.

A nominal group approach (Van de Ven and Delbecq, 1971) is used so that each member of the group (1) will have an *equal opportunity* to share information and (2) will be reinforced so that he or she will tend to share a *maximum amount* of relevant data. Facilitators can expect a degree of protest and resistance to the process by those members of the group accustomed to enjoying the lion's share of time in such a situation. On the other hand, the usually quiet group members often find this experience a very positive one. Maintaining a balance between these two responses is a primary skill required of the facilitator. This methodology specifically constrains group-process issues so that the group may most efficiently accomplish the task at hand: *the identification of priority problems that are maximally relevant to the represented constituencies of the organization.*

The time required to complete the above process in a workshop will vary between three and four hours. The authors have usually provided other types of activities in such workshops, including communication training, problem-solving skill development, team building, and others. Such activities can be mixed in effectively with the diagnostic activities. However, it is suggested that once the nominal group process begins that it not be interrupted until completed and group discussion has run its course.

Information *should not be shared among the different constituency groups* until after the priority problems have been developed independently. To do so would tend to "pollute" the uniqueness of the respective constituency information. Once each group has finished with the process, a sharing of these priority problems between constituencies is desirable and serves as a means of effectively ending the workshop.

If the workshop contains two or more stratified groups

from the same constituency, whose members are identical in characteristics, they should share their *present situation* data with each other before proceeding to the *desired situation* phase. In explanation, it is desirable to raise the awareness of all members of a particular constituency in relation to the *present situation* as much as possible. There is no need to keep the group separate to keep from mixing biases, since there are assumed to be no appreciable differences among the points of view of the groups in such cases. It is useful to allow the exchange of more information, earlier, to further stimulate member participation during the next step in the process. By so doing, the possibility of more creative and relevant *desired situations* is increased.

Experience and Application of Process Diagnosis

Experience in a number of situations has demonstrated the need to adhere to "rules" of the methodology. There must be some commitment on the part of the participants to want to examine their organizational problems. High information-holders must be selected as participants. Norms of sharing information, of allowing everyone "air time," of not evaluating until all information is given, and others must be established early to ensure that information is maximized and that the process moves along and does not stagnate. If any of these rules are not enforced, the group session can be particularly nonproductive and frustrating.

The methodology has been employed in many organizational interventions, including seven with community mental health centers. Problem diagnosis workshops were planned for each individual center. The workshops conducted with the centers produced much data for diagnosis of their organizational problems and provided insights into the methodology and the potential problems in its application. These mental health center workshops surfaced some particular problems encountered in the formation of two of the constituency groups: resource-providers and service-acquirers. These groups were difficult to organize because their membership consisted of individuals who were outside the organizational boundaries. In the case of service-acquirers, representatives from client community-service organizations tended to participate in the groups rather than individual clients of the center. This tendency might be attributed to the concern for client confidentiality in the mental health field. Also, considerable effort was required to demonstrate to potential group members that participation would be in their interest; this was particularly true in the case of resource-providers. In the end, the workshop had to be conducted without a resource-providers group, although we knew that the quality of the diagnosis would suffer without assembling all constituencies.

Another application of the methodology has also occurred in the data-gathering phases of a feasibility study for a Comprehensive Epilepsy Program. The four-constituency model was used to identify and group individuals as information sources and potential participants in a comprehensive program. Two organizational units were defined: the service component of the Comprehensive Epilepsy Program, and the research component of the program. The four constituencies for each component were defined and constituency groups were formed in recognition of the medical service/social service and urban/rural characteristics of the constituencies. A total of 12 groups was organized as a result. These workshops generated a large quantity of information that was useful in designing a comprehensive program.

Although the models and techniques described have been used most extensively in human-service delivery fields, numerous workshops have also been conducted with industrial clients. In these instances the full model has not been employed. Rather, different fragments of the two "internal" constituencies, technology-developers and direct-service providers, have been involved.

There is no apparent reason that the whole methodology could not be utilized in an industrial setting as it was in the human-service cases. For example, suppose a small manufacturing plant encountering personnel problems on the third shift asked for the services of a consultant. He or she might suggest that an organizational diagnosis be performed and explain the rationale for the method. The consultant would assist those within the organization retaining his/her services to identify the organizational unit (for example, production department-third shift) and the different constituencies involved in the situation. In this case, the manufacturing manager, the quality control manager, and the financial and sales personnel would be the resource-providers; the shift superintendent, the assistant shift superintendents, and the shift foremen would be technology-developers; the production workers on the third shift would be the direct-service providers; and the quality control inspectors and other personnel in receiving and shipping would be the service-acquirers. A determination might be made that it would be most appropriate to do an initial diagnosis with one group consisting of representatives from each constituency, particularly if the organizational unit is small. As suggested earlier, the composition would probably include two individuals per constituency. Individual constituency groups could be organized later as necessary. Negotiations would determine the extent to which the method should be employed. Deciding factors would include the acuteness of the pain felt by the members of the organization in its present situation and the commitment to the change process—or action—after the problems are defined.

Advantages of a Process-Oriented Organizational Diagnosis

The self-diagnostic process-oriented approach tends to overcome the disadvantages of the more conventional content-influential approaches in the following ways:

• The methodology encourages the client organization to produce its own information in the language that it best understands, and at no time are the data given up by the client. Each group owns its data and decides for itself what should be done with them in the future. This condition is insisted upon by the consultant from the outset of the intervention.

It has been the authors' experience that this norm is usually respected.

• The consultant is limited to influencing how information is collected in a way that is optimally relevant to the organization. The interventionist's values are excluded from the content of the data and a minimum of jargon is introduced.

• The process-oriented approach provides a qualitatively different procedure for diagnosis-feedback. Notice that the client role is changed from a *passive* one of information giving and receiving in relation to the interventionist to an *active* one in which the interventionist provides the *diagnostic process* by which the client system does its own generation and diagnosis of data. The consultant is constrained to emphasize process values over content values by the procedure.

• Not only is a basic organizational diagnosis accomplished with this methodology, but some specific issues related to collaborative processes are also *experienced*. It is quite common for group members to gain many initial insights into group process issues *without their being discussed* directly. The participants are placed in a situation where they experience problems of interpersonal communication rather than talk about such problems. They experience the contrast between support and nonsupport in a group situation, and between individual and group dimensions of the collaborative process as they intently engage the other members in their own self-chosen topics. All of these experiences can tend to reinforce a greater acceptance of a collaborative process and the development of collaborative skills. The tendency for the client to feel threatened by or dependent on the consultant is therefore minimized.

• The emphasis placed on the dichotomy of present situation/desired situation creates conditions that reinforce cognitive dissonance. In approaches that ignore *what is* and concentrate on *what has been* or *ought to be*, the level of dissonance is controlled. The process-oriented method we are describing, however, is designed to accentuate dissonance by first forcing the group members to concentrate on and describe the present. When emphasis is later given to the articulation of idealistic fantasies of the future, the contrast is accentuated and dissonance is reinforced. The listing of items about the present situation provides specificity about current conditions that can be used to stimulate an awareness of increased options in terms of the desired situation. The dissonance is an inherent product of this methodology which can provide the impetus needed for organizational members to commit themselves to other activities required in a change effort.

• The particular dynamic orientation of the problem definitions is also considered reinforcing to future change. In traditional approaches, problem definitions are rather static statements such as, "The problem is that we don't know what top management is doing," or, "The problem is that I don't have enough time to plan." In other words, typical problem statements are really statements of present situations. In the methodology we propose, the "problem defined" is *to change the present situation to the desired situation*. This is a much more dynamic—and realistic—orientation for effective problem-solving action.

After the Diagnosis . . .

The process-oriented diagnostic approach that is proposed here has been tested in many types of organizations. It has proven to be an effective way for an organization to engage in diagnosis, to accomplish awareness-raising with a minimum of conscious threat to the organization, and to provide for the kind of cognitive dissonance that can energize the organization to undergo change. A change effort that could follow from such a diagnosis would take these first steps:

1. All constituency groups identify restraining and driving forces that bear on movement from the present to the desired situation to further specify and identify factors pertaining to the organization's potential for change.

2. Action steps would be identified to remove forces that

tend to restrain the present situation from becoming the desired situation, and to assist forces that tend to drive the present situation to become the desired situation (Eisen, 1969).

3. The constituency groups would organize action teams that would *take action* for solving the priority problems.

Obviously, these steps are an oversimplification of a very difficult and complex process in organizational life. Diagnosis in itself does not ensure action or change, but it is an important first phase in organizational problem solving. Phases following the problem diagnosis phase, i.e., problem analysis, action planning, and action-taking phases, are being elaborated and will be described in future research reports.

At best, organizational change is difficult. It is suggested here that the first step toward effective change is to initiate an effective diagnosis of the organization (Bowers, 1973; Buchanan, 1971). For such an event to be maximally effective, the intervention should be as process oriented as possible, certain "rules" must be followed, and all of the important constituencies that influence the ultimate change processes in any organization should be included.

References and Readings

Alderfer, C., and Brown, R. Understand the impact of survey feedback. In W. W. Burke and H. Hornstein (Eds.), *The social technology of organization development.* Fairfax, Va.: NTL/Learning Resources Corporation, 1972.

Argyris, C. *Intervention theory and method: A behavioral science view.* Reading, Mass.: Addison-Wesley, 1970.

Bartee, E. A holistic view of problem solving. *Management Science*, 1973, 20 (4).

Bowers, D. OD techniques and their results in 23 organizations: The Michigan ICL Study. *Journal of Applied Behavioral Science*, 1973, 9, 21-43.

Bowers, D., and Franklin, J. Survey-guided development using human resources measurement in organizational change. *Journal of Contemporary Business*, 1972, 1, 43-55.

Buchanan, P. Crucial issues in OD. In H. A. Hornstein, B. B. Bunker, W. W. Burke, M. Gindes, and R. J. Lewicki (Eds.), *Social Intervention: A behavioral science approach*. New York: Free Press, 1971.

Crozier, M. *Le Phénomène Bureaucratique*. Paris: Editions du Seuil, 1963.

Dalton, G. Influence and organizational change. In G. Dalton and P. Lawrence (Eds.), *Organizational change and development*. Homewood, Ill.: Irwin-Dorsey, 1970.

Delbecq, A., and Van de Ven, A. A group process model for problem identification and program planning. *Journal of Applied Behavioral Science*, 1971, 7, 466-492.

Eisen, S. *A Problem-solving program for defining a problem and planning action*. Washington, D.C.: NTL Institute for Applied Behavioral Science, associated with The National Education Association, 1969.

Festinger, L. *A theory of cognitive dissonance*. New York: Row-Peterson, 1957.

Golembiewski, R. *Renewing organizations*. Itasca, Ill.: Peacock Publications, 1972.

Gorden, R. *Interviewing, strategy, techniques, and tactics*. Homewood, Ill.: Dorsey Press, 1969.

Greiner, L. Patterns of organizational change. *Harvard Business Review*, 1967, 45, 119-128.

Heyns, R., and Lippitt, R. Systematic observation techniques. In G. Lindsey (Ed.), *Handbook of social psychology*, Vol. 1. Reading Mass.: Addison-Wesley, 1954.

Klein, J. *Working with groups*. London: Hutchinson and Company, Ltd., 1966.

Levinson, H. *Organizational diagnosis.* Cambridge, Mass.: Harvard University Press, 1972.

Likert, R. *The human organization.* New York: McGraw-Hill, 1967.

Lorsch, L., and Lawrence, P. The diagnosis of organizational problems. In J. Thomas and W. Bennis (Eds.), *Management of change and conflict.* New York: Penguin Books, 1972.

Matarazzo, J., and Wiens, A. *The interview, research on its anatomy and structure.* Chicago: Aldine (Atherton), 1972.

Miles, M., Hornstein, H., Callahan, D., Calder, P., and Schiavo, R. The consequences of survey feedback: Theory and evaluation. In W. Bennis, K. Benne, and R. Chin (Eds.), *The planning of change,* 2nd ed. New York: Holt, Rinehart and Winston, 1969.

Neff, Frank W. Survey research: A tool for problem diagnosis and improvement in organizations. *Applied sociology.* New York: Free Press, 1965.

Peak, H. Attitude and motivation. In M. Jones (Ed.), *Nebraska Symposium on Motivation.* Lincoln: University of Nebraska, 1955.

Simon, H., and Newell, A. Human problem solving, the state of theory in 1970. *Proceedings of Annual Convention,* American Psychological Association, Miami, Florida, 1970.

Taylor, J., and Bowers, D. *Survey of organizations.* Ann Arbor: Institute for Social Research, University of Michigan, 1972.

Tichy, N., Hornstein, H., and Nisberg, J. Organization diagnosis and intervention strategies: Developing emergent pragmatic theories of change. Paper presented at the NTL Institute Conference on New Technology in Organization Development, New Orleans, February 1974.

Van de Ven, A., and Delbecq, A. Nominal versus interacting groups for committee decision-making effectiveness. *Journal of the Academy of Management,* 1971, 14 (2).

Zajonc, R., and Wolfe, D. Cognitive consequences of a person's position in a formal organization. *Human Relations*, 1966.

APPENDIX B

Seminar in
Mental Health Administration

Thomas Dolgoff
The Menninger Foundation

Seminars in Mental Health Administration

Topical Outline

A. Conceptions of Administration and Their Implications for Management

1. Definitions of Administration

   Purposes, persons and environments. Sources of administrative theory: economics, sociology, psychology, anthropology, political science.

2. Historical Outline of Administrative Theory

   The contributions of the pioneers. Recent contributions from the behavioral sciences: personality theory; interpersonal, group, and intergroup behavior.

3. Management Functions

   Planning, organizing, staffing, directing, coordinating, reporting, budgeting.

   Functional, metabolic, instrumental, expressive activities, "The Executive Role Constellation"; homeostatic, mediative, and proactive functions and avuncular-permissive, maternal-nurturant, and paternal-assertive roles.

   Managerial functions as relationships. Historical conceptions of the manager's job: father, teacher, counselor, overseer, decision maker. Relationships between administrators and governing boards: motivations and orientations, consumer representation.

   Clinician-executives and scientist-administrators: roles, functions, advantages, and problems.

4. Management Styles

   The continuum from autocratic to laissez faire management. Productive, receptive, exploiting, hoarding, and marketing executives. Likert's management diagnosis chart.

5. Management Skills

   Technical, human, conceptual, creative, innovative, conservative, and negotiating skills.

6. Group Processes in Administration

   Group norms. Characteristics of effective groups. Problems of individuals entering new groups, and their responses to resulting tensions. Task and group maintenance functions.

7. Management Myths

   One man—one boss. The manager as a supervisor. Management by results. Authority, responsibility, delegation. Participative management.

B. Motivation

1. Conceptions of Man and Their Implications for Management

   Beliefs as justifications for organizational behavior. Theories of man as self-fulfilling prophecies.

2. Rational-Economic Man

   Assumptions: hedonism, a fair day's work for a fair day's pay, men dislike work and must be motivated by economic incentives.

   Implications: emphasis on task performance, planning, organizing, controlling, close supervision.

3. Social Man

   Assumption: man is motivated by social needs.

   Implications: managers' expressive and instrumental functions; group processes, profit-sharing, fringe benefits.

4. Self-Actualizing Man

Assumptions: man's inherent need to use his skills and capacities; the manager as a catalyst and facilitator.

Implications: general supervision, contact and interaction, participative management, management by objectives, job enlargement.

5. Complex Man

Assumptions: Diversity, complexity, and inter-relationships of individual, interpersonal, group, and organizational goals. Differential needs for achievement, affiliation, and power. Psychoanalytic views of work motivation.

Implications: managerial flexibility and perceptiveness.

6. Personality and Organization (Argyris)

Discrepancies between human needs and organizational requirements and their consequences.

The hierarchy and the prepotency of needs. Criticisms of Argyris' and Maslow's theories.

7. The Psychological Contract (Levinson)

Dependence. Distance: affection, privacy, control. Change. Reciprocation.

8. Herzberg's Dual Theory of Motivation

Man's animal needs as dissatisfiers, "hygiene," or maintenance factors.

Man's human needs as motivators: to determine, achieve, discover, actualize, progress.

Implications: Intrinsic satisfactions in work, redesign of jobs to meet human needs. Job enlargement and job enrichment.

9. Motivations of Professionals in Organizations

Professional norms and values. Inter-professional and interdisciplinary conflict about purposes, methods, directions, roles, power, and status.

Strains between professionals and administrators in mental health agencies: Autonomy versus coordination, recruitment, supervision, patient and client screening, power and authority, innovation, rewards.

C. Power, Compliance, and Authority

1. Power

   Coercive, utilitarian, and normative power. Interactions between power-wielders and subjects.

   Power and decision: power, adjudication, and conflict management.

   Power and predictability: task performance, interdependence of parts, and social control.

   Other means of social control: environmental pressures, values, roles, and norms.

2. Compliance

   Alienation, compliance, and commitment in response to coercive, utilitarian, and normative power.

3. Typology of Organizations by Goals, Patterns of Power, Compliance, Reward, and Means of Control

4. Authority

   Authority as the legitimation of power and the basis for organizational structure. Group norms and peer pressure. Traditional, charismatic, structural, personal, and sapiential authority. The delegation of authority: authority, responsibility, accountability. Delegation as a problem of personality and personnel. Strategies and techniques for the delegation of authority. Organizational constraints.

5. Changing Concepts of Power and Authority

   Challenges to hierarchical models, military and ecclesiastical precedents, and the concept of "unity of command." Authority in American family life: immigration, technological change, and the obsolescence of parental wisdom. Limitations of various types of power: changes in dependency relationships of employer and employee, the symbolic meaning of material rewards, and changing moral codes.

6. Power and Authority in Professional Organizations

The expert's power of information, experience, and skill, and its limitations. The countervailing power of service groups and of pressures for coordination and control.

Power, uncertainty, and rules. Imbalance between ability and hierarchical power as a consequence of technological complexity and increased size and diversity.

7. Distinctive Problems in Mental Health Organizations

Problems in the exercise of authority: permissive and anti-authoritarian orientations. Delegation, the medical tradition, and professional norms.

Tensions between teams, disciplines, and service groups. Rules, the division of labor, and ambiguous technologies.

D. Organization

1. Definitions and Basic Concepts

Organization and authority, information, coordination, environment, and personality theory.

2. Characteristics of Effective Organizations

Self-renewal. Communication, structure, and climate.

3. Classifications of Organizations

Classification by power and compliance patterns: coercive, utilitarian, normative; by prime beneficiary: mutual benefit, business, service, commonweal; by transactions with the environment: interfaces between organization and environment, group and group, individual and organization, person and person.

Professional organizations. Autonomous and heteronomous professional organizations. Semiprofessional organizations.

4. Principles of Formal Organization

Task specialization: purpose, process, clientele, place. Segmentation in professional organizations.

Unity of command. Geographical, commodity, functional, departmentation.

Criteria for grouping activities. The exception principle: the locus and hierarchy of decision and authority.

Span of control, personal, personnel, economic, environmental, and intra-organizational factors. The scalar principle (chain of command).

Decentralization: technological and communication considerations. Impact of rules. Political factors.

Staff and line relationship: functions, authority, and responsibility of staff specialists and staff assistants. Reducing conflicts between staff and line officials. Staff and line concepts in professional organizations.

5. The Informal Organization

Friendship–kinship groups; cliques, subgroups, and isolates. Relation of formal and informal organization. Findings of the Hawthorne experiments. Social relationships, individual and group norms.

Functions of the informal organization for group satisfactions and stability; opportunities for social interaction, status, self-esteem, group acceptance, and leadership. The social organization of industry: jobs and pay as carriers of social values. Criticisms of the Hawthorne findings.

6. New Theories of Organization and Management

Likert's theories: The principle of supportive relationships, the role of the work group, linking-pin organization. Team management. Decentralization. Front-line administrators. Functional organization. Temporary organization.

E. **The Purpose and Nature of Supervision**

1. Supervision and Authority

   Clinical and administrative supervision. New concepts.

2. The Supervisee

   The supervisee's attitudes, needs, and values: self-concept, self-esteem, dependency needs, and attitudes towards change. Learning patterns in psychotherapy: the "Don Juans of psychotherapy," learning by denial, and submission.

   Determinants of upward communication. Functions of reports and records.

3. The Supervisor

   The supervisor's tasks: motivation, support, the exercise of authority. The supervisor's need for acceptance. Fostering dependency in supervisees. Clinical orientations in administrative settings.

   Determinants of effective supervision: listening, empathy, identification. The supervisor's boundary relationships as a source of role conflict. Instrumental and expressive leadership. Supervisory techniques: general and close supervision. Working supervisors. Separation of administrative and technical supervision.

4. Alternatives to Formal Supervision

   Advantages of discussion and consultation among colleagues: conformity to professional norms, reduced dependency, less information distortion, increased group cohesiveness.

   Disadvantages of nonfunctional informal hierarchies and differentiated informal statuses.

Functions of jokes or complaints about clients, patients, students.

Organizational arrangements.

5. Performance Appraisals

Purposes: inventory of skills, motivation, salary determinations, promotions and transfers.

Methods: performance versus personality, peer group comparisons, objectivity, counseling.

Evaluation of present methods: problems of raters and subordinates. Unintended effects on morale and performance.

Zero-sum problems in peer comparisons: displacement of goals.

Management by objectives as alternative to peer comparison ratings: open-ended, future-oriented, flexible.

Reports and auditing for performance appraisal. Tensions between auditors and managers. Unintended consequences of reports and audits: displacement of goals, inhibition of free communication, inadequacies of end result measures. Improving auditing and reporting procedures by participation, involvement, and horizontal rather than vertical feedback.

6. Job Enlargement

Job enlargement and motivation, knowledge, responsibility, growth, and advancement.

Methods of enlarging jobs: visibility of end results, inspection responsibilities, feedback to employees, participation in standard setting. "Optimal understaffing."

7. Management by Objectives

Relationships of tasks and goals. Personal style. Accountability for results rather than processes. The supervisor as a consultant. Organizational requirements: organizational values, flexibility, and training commitments.

Methods: Cost reduction versus profit-sharing. Group incentives versus individual incentives. Applications to nonprofit hospitals. Criticisms: Problems in end result measurement. Displacement of goals. Increased intergroup conflict.

8. Methods Improvement

Needs: rising costs, third-party payments, staff shortages.

Requirements: motivation, top management support, organizational climate.

Philosophy: effective problem-finding; employee participation. Techniques and tools: recognition, examination, evaluation, installation, follow-up. Process chart, flow diagram, organization chart, work distribution chart, procedure flow chart, work sampling.

Guidelines: Reduction of transcription and duplication of records. Statement of purposes of procedure guides. Costs and benefits of control mechanisms.

Illustrations: accounting and billing, admission and bed control, dietary, housekeeping, mail, maintenance, medical records, nursing, reports.

F. Decision

1. Definitions

Decision, facts, values, and choice.

2. Conditions Needed for Sound Decisions

Definition of the problem. Distinctions between means and ends. Search for alternatives and study of consequences. Limits of rationality: values, perceptions, capacities. Selection of solutions. Nonrational factors: intuition, judgement, personality factors, role ambiguity and conflict, selective perception, false analogies.

3. Group Decision Making

Decision by nonresponse, authority, majority rule, minority, consensus, unanimous consent. Group decisions and "the technostructure." Problem solving by committees.

4. Decision and Organization

Decision and hierarchy. The authority of ideas and of sanctions.

5. Decisions, Power, and Authority

Executives as ratifiers. The premises of decision.

6. Policy and Executive Element in Decision

Optimizing and balancing. Maintaining stability within governing relationships. "Appreciation," judgement, decision.

G. Communication

1. Definitions

Language, information, and sentiments. Nonverbal communication: gestures, posture, actions, symbols, kinesics.

2. Importance of Communication

Effects on planning, organizing, and coordinating in the formal organization.

Effects on motivation, morale, and emotional climate in the informal organization.

3. Barriers to Effective Communication

Ambiguity of purpose. Semantic problems: meanings of words, contexts, frames of reference. Filtering in interpersonal communications: effects of hierarchical structure, power advantages, perception of self and others, feelings, attitudes, and expectations.

4. Self-Fulfilling Prophecies in Communication

The atmosphere of the organization. Levels of communication: latent and manifest messages. The parts of a person: the open self, the concealed self, the blind self, the unknown self.

5. How Communications Can Be Improved

    Attitudes and skills of communicators. Training. The clarity and medium of the message. The capacities and readiness of the recipient. Identifying possible unintended consequences. Informal pretesting. Skill in listening.

H. Introducing Change

1. The Need for Change

    Environmental factors—economic and technological. Internal factors: personnel, research and training, physical plant and location. Operating deficiencies, vested interests. Effects of failure to change.

2. Resistance to Change

    Perseverance of habit and custom. Threats to security and status. Fear of the unfamiliar.

3. Conditions Necessary for Successful Change

    Experience of stress. Authority and power of initiators. Coalitions.

4. Reducing Resistance to Change

    Conditions necessary for acceptance of orders. Coherence of message. Receivers' capacities, self-interest, and perception of organizational goals. Demonstrated advantages to those affected. Recognized limitations of rationality.

    Assess possible unintended consequences on formal and informal organization, established policies and procedures, and personal goals and values.

    Recognize importance of timing: the context of change, pilot programs, limited commitments.

Secure participation of those affected in planning and execution.

Match the change method to the type and amount of change desired: differential strategies for changes in interaction, role expectations, orientations and values, and basic motives. Cognitive and emotional elements in change.

Strategies in mental health agencies: linkages, versatility of staff, job rotation, social relationships. Rationale and justification for radical and rapid change.

Contraindications to participation.

I. Conflict and Conflict Management

1. Values and Costs of Conflict

   Motivation and energy because of heightened sense of necessity. Self-understanding because of need to articulate views. Psychological values for the managing of internal needs and conflicts.

   Organizational advantages for vitality and identification of problem areas.

   Negative consequences for individuals, groups, task performance, communication and morale.

   Common stresses of executives: status and competition anxiety; fear of failure; guilt at success.

2. Role Conflict

   Conflicts between internal standards of value and the defined role behavior. Conflicting expectations from one person. Incompatible expectations from two or more persons. Role overload and conflict in priorities.

   Organizational factors: Problems and misunderstandings across organizational boundaries. Tensions between instrumental and expressive leadership. The foreman as the "master and victim of doubletalk." Conflicts between innovators and conservators. Mobility aspirations and frustrations of middle managers. Employees' defenses against anxiety-provoking task requirements. Conflicts between professionals and administrators.

Personality factors: Emotional sensitivity and neurotic anxiety. Introversion-extroversion, flexibility-rigidity, and needs for career achievement.

Interpersonal factors: Organizational interdependence and role stress. Formal role relations and informal interpersonal conflicts and bonds.

Interaction of organizational, personality, and interpersonal factors. Core problems and derivative problems. The costs of coping maneuvers and their unintended consequences.

Consequences of role conflict: job dissatisfaction, cognitive and emotional disturbances, withdrawal and projection of blame.

Alleviation of role conflict. Structural change, specialized liaison positions, "promotive interdependence," personnel selection and placement, training in group dynamics.

3. Role Ambiguity and Status Inconsistency

Determinants of role ambiguity: supervisors' evaluations, opportunities for advancement, scope of responsibility, expectations of performance.

Sources of role ambiguity. Complexity of tasks, rapidity of change, inter-relatedness of roles, restriction of information.

The functions and symbols of status: Formal and informal status. The status system and organizational and psychological needs, incentives, and satisfactions. Rank, privileges, and obligations as status symbols.

Status inconsistency: Social and occupational distance. Differences in status on and off the job. Conflicts when demands flow contrary to status lines.

4. Interpersonal Conflict

Definitions: Substantive issues such as competition for resources, philosophical differences, role invasion, task deprivation. Emotional issues such as personal need deprivation, incompatible personal needs, differences in personal style.

Barriers to conflict or to conflict resolution: attitudes, values, needs, fears, and habits. Group norms, time limitations, fears of nonresponse to conciliation, physical barriers.

Triggering events: decision on policies, resource allocations, opportunities for advancement.

Conflict tactics: blocking, interrupting, depreciating, forming alliances, injecting substantive issues into emotional conflicts, adding derivative issues.

5. Inter-Group Conflict

Types of group conflict in organizations: functional conflicts between production, maintenance, regulatory and managerial subsystems. The power tactics of service groups which control scarce resources. Direct competition between similar subsystems. Hierarchical conflict over organizational rewards.

Consequences of inter-group competition: group climate, task orientation, and leadership patterns before and after decision. Consequences to winners and losers.

6. Inter-Organization Conflict

Organizations in competition. Organizations performing complementary functions.

7. Conflict Management and Resolution

Distinctions between conflict management and conflict resolution. Suppression, total war, limited war, bargaining, problem solving.

The management of interpersonal conflict: Preventing

ignition of a conflict interchange by blunting triggering events. Constraining the form of the conflict by limiting weapons and tactics, invoking group norms, and providing extra-organizational supports for consequences of conflict.

Advantages and disadvantages of confrontation. Inhibitions to confrontation. Confrontation strategies and incentives: achieving balance in situational power, synchronizing confrontation efforts, the pacing of dialogues, improving communication reliability, maintaining optimum tension.

The management of inter-group conflicts: Changes in personnel practices, roles, and organizational arrangements within existing systems. Developing additional machinery for conflict adjudication, such as grievance procedures and arbitration. Restructuring the organization to reduce built-in conflict by linking-pin organization, changes in the locus of decision, decentralization, changes in reward systems, job enlargement and enrichment, and management by objectives.

8. Distinctive Processes and Problems in Mental Health Agencies

Competition for resources related to segmentation along lines of professional interests and incompatibility of professional norms.

Integration through political processes. Alliances based on differential status, needs, and ideologies.

The effects of graduate school education on the norms of "the free professional" in an organizational setting.

J. Organizations As Open Systems

1. History and Viewpoints of System Theory

The fusing of mechanistic and organismic approaches to the unification of science. Purpose and goal-seeking behavior as related to physical processes. Distinctions between inanimate and animate nature.

Recent developments in system theory: cybernetics, gestalt psychology, communication theory, decision theory. Open system theory and psychiatry: Mental illness as disorganization. The ego as an advanced subsystem. Analogies between the ego and the manager, and between psychopathology and organizational ineffectiveness.

2. Basic Concepts

Static and dynamic systems and subsystems. Closed and open systems. Input, throughput, output.

Functions and permeability of boundaries. System openness. Physical and psychological boundaries.

Coding mechanisms: selective perception and response, positive and negative feedback.

Negative entropy in biological and social systems. The steady state and dynamic homeostasis. Differentiation. Equifinality: initial conditions and final states in open and closed systems, and in mechanical and organismic systems.

3. Distinctive Characteristics of Organizations as Open Systems

Organizations as problem-solving systems mediating competing demands for stability and change, and for the processing of information.

Organizations as social systems which structure events rather than physical parts. Psychological structure. Roles, norms, and values as organizational cement.

Formalized role systems to define interdependent behavior and enforce rules. Partial inclusion as the basis for bureaucratic organization. Consequences for the manager's instrumental and expressive functions.

System norms and values: organizational loyalty, the norm of reciprocity, organizational culture and climate.

Organizational space: geographical, functional, and hierarchical.

System dynamic. Motivational forces of systems and subsystems as related to task requirements, opportunities, constraints, and clientele. Acquisitive and extractive mechanisms as common dynamics.

4. Functions, Dynamics, and Mechanics of Organizational Subsystems

Production subsystems and the dynamic of efficiency.

Supportive subsystems for material procurement and product disposal, and the dynamic of environmental relationships.

Maintenance subsystems for staff recruitment and socialization and the dynamic of stability and conservation.

Adaptive subsystems for research, development and planning, and the dynamic of change.

Managerial subsystems for regulatory mechanisms and the authority structure. The dynamics of control, compromise, survival, and growth.

K. Constraints on Organizational Effectiveness

Organizational shells of survival, stability, purpose, and membership and resistance to change.

1. Need for Stability

Innovations as threats to equilibrium. Social relationships and fear of change. Personal threat in criticisms of current practice. Local pride as an inhibitor. Inertia. Socialization of new members to accept old ways.

2. Coding Scheme Barriers

Common coding schemes and unique vocabularies. Blocking and distortion of needed information. Fear of malevolence of outsiders. Status differences among systems, subsystems, and their interaction.

3. Economic Conditions, Experimentation, and Risk

4. Goal Definition and Restriction of Output

5. Displacement of Goals

   Vested interests, fixation on internal problems, co-optation of opposition, confusion of means and ends in subsystems and larger systems.

6. Goal Conflict

   Conflicts in goals, norms, needs, and values of individuals, groups, and organizational subsystems and dispersion of energy.

   Disagreements about values and methods. "The Discontent Explosion in Mental Health."

7. Division of Labor, Hierarchy, and Differential States

   Division of labor, perceptual distortion, and interunit competition.

   Hierarchy, differential status, and blockage to communication flow.

   Roles and pressure for conformity.

   Bennis' critique of bureaucracy.

   Bureaucratic organization in psychiatric hospitals: roles, impersonality, technological difficulties, multiple subordination.

8. Span of Control and Dependency

9. Centralization and Conformity

10. Delegation of Authority

    Delegation as a problem of personality, personnel, and structure.

    The traditions of medical practice.

    "The state of the art" and delegation and performance standards in psychiatry.

11. Imbalance between Ability and Authority

12. Leadership Behavior

13. Informal Organization
    Functions.
    Informal organizations in mental health agencies.

14. Professionalism
    Professional norms, "encroachment," and conflicts among professional groups.
    Conflict and innovation. Segmentation in professional organizations.

15. Teams versus Disciplines in Mental Health Agencies
    Limitations on the power and authority of interdisciplinary team leaders.
    Functions and power strategies of teams and disciplines.
    Negotiation in mental health agencies.

16. Characteristics of Staff in Mental Health Agencies
    Superspecialization, blocked mobility, and differential status.
    Performance and personality.
    Effects of conflict on patient behavior.

L. Strategies for the Improvement of Organizational Effectiveness in Mental Health Agencies

1. Environmental Constraints, Pressures, and Opportunities Contributing to Organizational Effectiveness
   Competition and perception of crises as incentives to change. Organizational invaders entering a safe and stable market. Goal succession, multiplication, and expansion when old goals have been met or cannot be attained.

2. Linkage
   The number and variety of interpersonal, inter-group,

and inter-organizational connections; interrelatedness, reciprocal and collaborative relationships between resource systems and user systems.

Examples: Members with strong professional ties who strengthen the organization while advancing their profession. Overlapping groups and the organizational linking of supervisors and subordinates horizontally and vertically.

3. Openness

Flexibility and accessibility. Optimal permeability of system and subsystem boundaries. Belief that change is possible and desirable. Willingness to give and receive outside help and to listen to others. Social climate favorable to change.

Examples: Awareness of external resources, the use of consultants and change agents. The training of supervisors in group dynamics and human relations. Work group relationships which encourage open expression of feelings and needs. The encouragement of constructive conflict and its management.

4. Capacity

The capability to marshal diverse resources: wealth, power, size, centrality, intelligence, education, experience, versatility.

Examples: Change in leadership which brings new perspectives and knowledge. Skill and versatility of the staff with the technical, human, and conceptual skills pertinent to their tasks.

5. Reward

The frequency, immediacy, amount, and mutuality of positive reinforcements. Material, social, and symbolic rewards and incentive plans. Professional as well as administrative career ladders.

6. Proximity

Nearness in time, place, and context. Familiarity, similarity, recency.

7. Structure

Effective and function division of labor and coordination of effort. Systematic planning and execution. Integration of technological, psycho-social, maintenance, regulatory, adaptive, and managerial subsystems.

General strategies, including internal knowledge-seeking units, specialized output roles and subsystems, wide participation in planning and decision, decentralization and reduction in organizational levels.

Specific strategies for mental health agencies including interdisciplinary teams, clinician-executive roles, first-line administrators as linking-pins, temporary organization.

Organizations as socio-technical systems in which technical, psycho-social, and structural subsystems are in synergistic interaction.

8. Synergy

The number, variety, frequency, and persistence of forces that can be mobilized. Continuity and synchronization of effort.

APPENDIX C

Example of Developing
Learning Objectives upon Which
Evaluations May Be Based

Reprinted from *Guidelines and Standards for Professional Master's Degree Programs in Public Affairs/Public Administration*, by permission of the National Association of Schools of Public Affairs and Administration.

	Knowledge	Skills	Values	Behavior
Political-Social-Economic Context	1. Cultural and social mores and patterns 2. Political values and processes 3. Economic systems, incentives and controls 4. Governmental institutions, powers and relationships 5. Environmental factors and resource availabilities	1. Analysis and interpretation of political-social-economic forces and trends 2. Application of political-social-economic knowledge to solution of public problems 3. Evaluation of the political-social-economic impact and consequences of administrative policies and actions	1. Democratic traditions and practices, constitutionalism and the rule of law 2. The purposes and limitations of government as an instrument for fostering social and economic progress 3. Access for individuals and groups to centers of power and decision making 4. The political direction and responsibility of administration and administrators 5. Standards of official/personal conduct and ethics	1. Tolerance of diverse views of other persons and groups 2. Capacity to adjust to complex political-social environments and situations 3. Ability to function as a social organizational change agent 4. Participation in public action programs, e.g., community development projects, citizen advisory groups etc.
Analytical Tools: Quantitative and Nonquantitative	1. Quantitative decision methodology, e.g., accounting, parametric and nonparametric statistics, linear programming, modeling, etc.	1. Logical analysis and diagnosis 2. Research design and application 3. Computer utilization and application 4. Application of quantitative and nonquantitative methodology to organizational situations	1. Objectivity and rationality in the conduct of public affairs 2. Utilization of science and research to foster public purposes	1. Involvement in data gathering and problem-solving exercises 2. Familiarity with public documents, legal sources, and form of administrative communications

111

Knowledge	Skills	Values	Behavior
2. Electronic data processing and information systems 3. Systems and procedures analysis; e.g., organization surveys, work measurement, etc.	5. Oral and written communications and presentations	3. Impartial inquiry and investigation of public needs and problems 4. Openness in communication and interpretation of data and findings to the public	3. Preparation of correspondence, reports, and position papers 4. Participation in professional associations, internships, and other forms of experiential learning
Individual/Group/Organizational Dynamics 1. Individual and group behavior e.g., individual motivation, dynamics of groups, modes of leadership, etc. 2. Organization structure, process dynamics, e.g., models, authority, development strategies, decision making, etc. 3. Communications theory and process 4. Professionalism and public service, e.g., evolution of public services, roles and standards of professions, characteristics of bureaucracies, etc.	1. Personal motivation and leadership 2. Interpersonal and group relationships 3. Identification and analysis of political and organizational power 4. Application of appropriate models of organization, leadership, and decision making 5. Coping with organizational stresses, limitations, and change	1. Protection and fostering of individual rights, liberties, and welfare 2. Promotion of organizational equity and effectiveness 3. Reconciliation of private interests with public objectives and needs 4. Concern for the clients served by the organization	1. Consistency, genuineness and integrity in human and organizational relationships 2. Positive attitudes concerning individual growth and organizational improvement 3. Willingness to share insights and experiences with others 4. Recognition and understanding of variations in human and organizational motivations and approaches

Policy Analysis	1. Application of analytical and administrative tools to solution of public problems 2. Processes by which policy is formulated, implemented, and evaluated 3. Strategies for optimization and selection of alternatives 4. Distinctive attributes of policy relative to specific functional areas, e.g., health, transportation, etc.	1. Socio-economic analysis, e.g., cost benefit analysis, social impact analysis, etc. 2. Political diagnosis, e.g., public opinion evaluation, group power surveys, legislative-executive relationships, etc. 3. Problem comprehension and interpretation, e.g., identification of strategic issues, liaison skills, advocacy, etc. 4. Policy measurement, scaling, and design 5. Program impact measurements, e.g., program evaluation, outcome or effectiveness measurement, etc.	1. The use of data and analysis to enlarge the scope of public choice 2. Policies and programs which foster equality of opportunity and well-being 3. Measures to increase citizen understanding of public policies and their impact 4. Standards of program formulation and conduct 5. Procedures for full and fair assessment of program benefits and costs to various publics 6. Measures to increase client and public participation in public policy formulation and evaluation	5. Participation in professional associations, internships and other forms of experiential learning 1. Ability to relate and integrate diverse factors to common objectives 2. Methods of adaptation to political and organizational pressures and constraints 3. Ability to bargain, compromise, and arbitrate 4. Participation in professional associations, internships, and other forms of experiential learning

Administrative/Management Processes	Knowledge	Skills	Values	Behavior
	1. Administrative planning and organizational design	1. Conceptualizing, goal setting, organization design and program development	1. The role and use of organizations and administrative processes to achieve public objectives	1. Openness to new ideas and proposals
	2. Management systems and processes including leadership, decision making, direction, and organization development and change	2. Work assignment and supervision	2. Standards of efficiency and effectiveness in the conduct of the public's business	2. Recognition and consideration of strengths, weaknesses, and desires of others
	3. Personnel administration, including staffing, training, and collective bargaining	3. Negotiating and persuading	3. Standards of individual and organizational integrity and performance	3. Facility in applying management tools and processes to varied organizational settings and problems
	4. Finance and budgeting	4. Monitoring, assessment, and review	4. Public surveillance and review by citizens and their elected representatives	4. Effectiveness in undertaking organization and management surveys
	5. Program evaluation and control		5. A working environment conducive to individual fulfillment and the attainment of public confidence	5. Participation in professional associations, internships, and other forms of experiential learning

114

APPENDIX D

Overview:
Management Training Program
William Garove and Thomas Fernekes

Management Training Program
Center for Developmental
and Learning Disorders

University of Alabama in Birmingham

The Management Training Program

Welcome to the Management Training Program. We are pleased to have you as a participant. Our program is specifically designed for management personnel employed in state residential and community-based facilities for the mentally retarded. Its training capabilities have been broadened to include university students with career potential or aspirations toward employment in a mental retardation facility. Conducted at the Center for Developmental and Learning Disorders, University of Alabama in Birmingham, it is the only continuing education program of its kind in the United States.

The program lasts one year and has three phases: two one-week, on-campus training seminars at the University of Alabama in Birmingham; a three-day site visit to a mental retardation facility; and eight comprehensive home study assignments.

Our program has been funded and sponsored since July 1, 1970 by HEW Region IV, Department of Social and Rehabilitation Services, Division of Developmental Disabilities. It also receives state fiscal support in that efforts are made to adhere to a 50 percent state and 50 percent Federal fiscal matching for participant travel and per diem expenses.

Although funded through HEW Region IV, our program serves seventeen states: Alabama, Arkansas, Delaware, Florida, Georgia, Kansas, Kentucky, Louisiana, Maryland, Mississippi, North Carolina, Oklahoma, South Carolina, Tennessee, Texas, Virginia, and West Virginia. Participants represent more than thirty different position classifications including superintendents, assistant superintendents, business managers, directors of in-service training, social services, psychology, cottage life, and nursing services. Educational backgrounds range from bachelor's to doctoral degrees from a wide variety of disciplines.

Purpose and Need

The *purpose* of our Management Training Program is to

117

improve individual management performance, organization of MR programs, and service-delivery systems. By improving your managerial proficiency through training, you should be better able to meet your professional responsibility of providing the best possible services to retarded people. A purpose must result from an identified need. There is a need for management training because:

1. As a manager, you are responsible for accomplishing organization objectives through human and material resources.
2. There is a lack of college and university programs that train management personnel to work in community-based and residential mental retardation facilities.
3. Inadequacies in the care and treatment of the retarded is related to ineffective institution management. This statement is supported by the AAMD Standards Report of 1965 and the 1968 Report of the President's Committee on Mental Retardation.
4. Management personnel of facilities for the retarded have frequently failed to recognize and apply training methods and management practices used successfully by business, industry, and other professions.
5. In-service management training is needed to avoid professional obsolescence, the failure of a once capable professional to achieve currently expected results. Twenty years in a management position should add up to twenty years of experience, not one year of experience twenty times.
6. Historically, people working as managers of mental retardation facilities come from such professional and academic backgrounds as psychology, social work, medicine, education, and others. Frequently, these backgrounds have not included training in basic management concepts or functions such as labor relations, budget and finance, personnel relations, public relations, plant planning, and organizational development.

118

Instructional Logic

With the purpose and need for the program specified, attention is directed to its instructional logic, basic objectives, and a description of the instructional format designed to meet those objectives. Both the instructional objectives and program activities are based on an identifiable systematic logic. This logic is Socratic in nature and designed to develop the participants' knowledge of:

- themselves as managers
- management—an operational definition; its development and basic concepts, such as planning, organizing, directing, controlling, coordinating, communicating, motivating, and decision making; and other salient functions, including labor relations, public relations, budget and finance, and plant planning
- others, interpersonal relationships with subordinates and superordinates
- MR facilities—background, development and organization, programs, and service delivery systems
- mentally retarded people—number, types, rights, and social influences regarding care, treatment, and education
- issues, trends, and innovations in mental retardation and management
- ways to apply accepted management principles, theories, and practices to the management of MR programs and facilities

Program Objectives

This systematic logic has been applied to the construction of a series of program objectives from which the content of the program evolved. These objectives are:

1. To increase your managerial proficiency through participation in a training program based on a systematic logic, accepted management principles, well-constructed objectives, and validated participant needs.

119

2. To provide a mechanism for you to develop a realistic perception of your management style.
3. To provide opportunities for you to assess your managerial performance and have your performance analyzed by fellow trainees and management instructors.
4. To provide you with opportunities to link management theory and practice through the use of simulation and other reality-based training techniques.
5. To provide you with the opportunities to learn and apply more effective individual and group problem-solving and decision-making skills.
6. To sensitize you to problems encountered by superintendents, directors, and other management personnel employed in residential and community-based facilities for the mentally retarded.
7. To provide opportunities for you to learn and apply accepted management principles, theories, and practices to the management of a simulated mental retardation facility and your facility.
8. To provide you with opportunities to develop your interpersonal and group relationship skills through the use of specific organization development and simulation exercises.
9. To provide you with specific methods for implementing systems changes within your own organizations, i.e., organizational structure, planning, employee appraisal, position descriptions, and others.

Instructional Content

Because a good instructional system requires constant analysis and evaluation, the program content is continually being revised and refined so it will meet the program objectives. Feedback from participants and consultation with our faculty and Advisory Committee have resulted in many improvements in the training program.

The theoretical content of the program is presented in the

120

first and final week seminars. Following is a list of the curriculum topics presented in these seminars and a brief description of the content of each:

FIRST WEEK SEMINAR

1. *Managerial Grid Theory.* Provides you with a theoretical framework within which you can identify and analyze your own style of management and the effect of five basic styles of management on accomplishing organization goals.
2. *Decision Making.* Presents you with a system designed to improve your individual decision-making ability and prove the value of group consensus decision making. This system can be adapted to the existing procedures for making decisions within any organization.
3. *Basic Concepts of Management.* Provides you with an operational definition of management and an explanation of the primary functions of management: planning, organizing, controlling, motivating, and communicating.
4. *Labor Relations.* Analyzes the history of unions and their impact on management and management styles. This information should help you to accept evidence which indicates that positive management-union relationships can evolve from a three-stage process of conflict, compromise, and cooperation.
5. *Organization Climates.* Presents information and strategies designed to improve your ability to anticipate and respond to external influences which affect you and your organization, i.e., parent groups, litigation, legislation, labor organization, innovations and trends, and new philosophies.
6. *Interpersonal Relationships.* Analyzes participant attitudes and opinions on what motivates people and compares them to the Herzberg Theory of Motivation. In addition, basic communication theory is explained and applied to the problem of employee morale in an organization.

121

7. *Management Organization and Job Descriptions.* Presents information which describes traditional organization structure as a tool of management and explains the need for clear, specific job descriptions within that organization structure.

8. *Legal Aspects of Mental Retardation.* Presents current information on the issues of both the legal and human rights of the mentally retarded. The intent is to give you a better understanding of your professional responsibilities as influenced by legal aspects of mental retardation.

FINAL WEEK SEMINAR

1. *Fundamentals of Financial Accounting.* Directed primarily to the manager with no accounting background, this component is designed to increase your knowledge and skills in the use of accounting as an organization control mechanism. Emphasis is also placed on the role of the accountant on the management team.

2. *Program Evaluation and Review Technique (PERT).* Provides you with a management tool which will improve your ability, as a manager, to plan, control, and evaluate programs within your organization.

3. *Principles of Budget Preparation.* Presents information intended to give you a better understanding of budgets and the budgeting process with particular attention given to defining and describing Planning, Programming, Budgeting System (PPBS), and Zero Based Budgets.

4. *Employee Counseling and Performance Appraisal.* Presents a system of organization which incorporates employee job descriptions, standards of performance for those job descriptions, and an employee appraisal system based on those performance standards. You will analyze traditional performance appraisal systems practices and learn techniques for employee counseling.

5. *Public Relations: Principles and Practices.* For instructional purposes, this presentation is divided into two parts: Part One analyzes the communication of information within the organization; Part Two analyzes the communi-

cation of information to the public through the news media. Emphasis is placed on having you learn that public relations is a part of every manager's job and that "PR" activities should be based on meeting your organization's objectives.

6. *Alternatives to Institutionalization.* Provides you with an opportunity to listen to and ask questions of a person, selected by the Management Training Program, who is knowledgeable in planning and implementing alternative service delivery systems for the mentally retarded.

7. *Effective Written Communications.* Presents material and information designed to help you produce written communications that are clear, concise, correct, and interesting.

8. *Computer Utilization by Management.* Presents nontechnical information about computers and their use. This information is applied specifically to problems related to managing service systems for the mentally retarded.

SIMULATION

The *Shannon State School and Hospital Simulator* is an important part of the training provided in the first and final week seminars. At the beginning of the first week, you are introduced to the "Shannon Materials" and the basic theory of simulation and how it is used to link theory and practice. You will view slide-tape presentations on Shannon State School and Hospital and on the community of Shannon. This information provides the context for the simulation exercises used throughout the program. You will assume the role of Superintendent of the simulated Shannon State School and Hospital. This role gives you the opportunity to apply the basic management theory and principles taught in the program to practical situations encountered in the management of a mental retardation facility.

Following the introduction to Shannon and your role as Superintendent, you begin simulation exercises. These exercises consist of in-basket items, live encounter items, and

123

telephone calls. In-basket items are letters, memos, and telephone messages. Live encounter items are contacts by telephone and personal visits.

In-basket items are used in team and individual simulation exercises. Team simulation sensitizes you to the types of problems presented in the simulator and introduces team management, a concept emphasized throughout the program. It provides the opportunity to practice making decisions and establishing priorities by group consensus. Additional sets of in-baskets are used in individual simulation exercises which give you the chance to "go it alone."

You are also responsible for processing at least two live encounter items. These are video-taped meetings between you, as Superintendent, and one or more other people. Encounters usually include a telephone interruption putting you in the position of handling two separate problems at the same time—not an uncommon predicament for managers. Encounters are designed to provide experiences relevant to improving your ability to manage. Anxiety or embarrassment is avoided by ensuring that you have the necessary resources to manage the problem presented. "Soap opera" crises and unsolvable problems have no place in the Shannon Simulator!

Group discussion on participant responses follows each simulation training exercise. Instructors generate discussion by using open-ended questions specifically designed to have you: (1) express the rationale for your decisions, (2) determine alternative solutions and explore their consequences, and (3) develop insight into your own managerial behavior. Instructors also use these post-simulation discussions to link management theory taught in the program to the practical situations presented in the simulations.

ORGANIZATION DEVELOPMENT

In addition to simulation, you will participate in structured organization development experiences during the first and final week seminars. These exercises are done in low-risk conditions. Because the training program emphasizes the team approach to management, OD exercises play an important part in analyzing your overt behavior and feelings during team-building and consensus-judgement activities. These exercises also help develop awareness of factors that are either barriers or facilitators to team effectiveness.

The instructional content of the Management Training Program's first and final week seminars provides you with useful methods of management taken from various disciplines and professions. The instructional activities of the program are based on specific behavioral objectives and presented using modern instructional materials and techniques, applied accepted management practices to current developments in mental retardation programming. And these instructional activities are tied together through the use of Shannon State School and Hospital Simulator and organization development exercises designed to link management theory and practice.

Following is a list of the first and final week instructional modes, the number of uses, and the time allocated to each:

Mode	Number	Time
Simulation	14	$18^1/_2$ hrs.
Lecture	20	$23^1/_4$ hrs.
Films	5	$2^1/_2$ hrs.
Slide-Tape	6	2 hrs.
Displays	1	$^1/_2$ hr.
Inventories, Tests	2	$2^1/_4$ hrs.
Discussions, Demonstrations, and Applications	11	$10^3/_4$ hrs.
Structured Organization Development Experiences	8	$10^1/_2$ hrs.
Assignments	4	4 hrs.
Miscellaneous	5	$4^1/_2$ hrs.
		$78^3/_4$ hrs.

HOME STUDY ASSIGNMENTS #1, #2, and #3

Following the first week seminar, approximately one year's

125

time passes before you return for your second week seminar. During this period you are required to complete eight home study assignments. Listed below are the first three assignments which provide a follow-up and reinforcement of the content presented in the first week seminar:

Assignment #1 Multiple choice exercise—questions intended to reinforce the learning of information taught during the first week seminar.

Assignment #2 Employee Appraisal System Manual—two position descriptions with standards of performance are applied to the participant's work situation.

Assignment #3 Labor Relations—development of a contingency plan for a union-precipitated emergency, and an explanation of the grievance procedures used at the participant's institution.

These three assignments are to be completed *before* you participate in the site visit.

SITE VISIT

Midway through your training year you will make a site visit to a residential mental retardation facility. This training activity is designed to (1) develop ongoing communications among management persons from various mental retardation facilities; (2) disseminate information about innovative and effective mental retardation programs; and (3) identify and analyze aspects of the host facility's organization structure and programs which are of relevance to your mental retardation facility. You then have the opportunity to apply the knowledge gained to the modification or development of your organization and its programs.

HOME STUDY ASSIGNMENT #4

While on the site visit you will complete Home Study Assignment #4—Site Visit Analysis. Completed home study assignments on the site visit are synthesized into a report which is given to and reviewed with the superintendent and other management staff of the site facility. The report is an objective compilation of participants' observations of the facility's organization, procedures, and programs. Feedback in the report is *exclusive* of affective judgments of individual personalities and performance, and is *not* an evaluation of the facility's program effectiveness.

HOME STUDY ASSIGNMENTS #5, #6, #7, AND #8

During the second half of your training year you are responsible for four additional home study assignments which introduce the content presented in the final week seminar. Because this introductory information is essential to the content of the final week seminar, you are required to complete and submit these four assignments before returning for your final week seminar.

Assignment #5   Programmed Evaluation Review Technique (PERT)—use of a programmed instruction book and an application of PERT to a real situation in participant's own facility.

Assignment #6   Principles of Public Relations—emphasis on the development of an effective PR program using all types of news media.

Assignment #7   Issues, Trends, Problems, and Innovations in Mental Retardation—use of a short answer essay format requiring an awareness of a variety of topics considered essential in the management of a mental retardation facility.

Assignment #8   Budgeting and Accounting—emphasis on basic budgeting and accounting principles for participants with no previous experience in these important management areas.

The Management Training Program uses two alternate assignments which accommodate circumstances where one of the required assigments may be of limited value to you in your work situation. For example, participants employed in small community-based mental retardation facilities have found the assignment on "Labor Relations" of limited use because the likelihood of unionization is remote. Consequently, one of the following alternate assignments may be chosen. Alternate Assignment #1, *Principles of Management*, is a programmed instruction text which provides an overview of the management concepts. It can be used as an introduction or a review of the management concepts taught throughout the program. Alternate Assignment #2, "Multiple Choice Learning Exercise," consists of questions prepared by each of the program's faculty members. These questions introduce the instructional content of the final week seminar. Alternate Assignment #3, *Introduction to Data Processing*, is a programmed instruction text which will provide you with information on computerized information retrieval and dissemination. This assignment will help you gain more from the presentation on "Computer Utilization by Management" in the final week seminar. Feedback on all home study assignments is provided by the Program's faculty within a month after the assignment is completed and submitted.

Summary

As the MTP expands and matures, the need to develop and implement selection criteria and performance standards for participants has become essential. Criteria for participant selection are needed to better identify people who would benefit from management training and are highly motivated to complete the program once they enroll. Proper selection procedures should ensure that the maximum number of people who begin the program will complete it.

Meeting clearly delineated standards of performance is a contemporary concept. Everyone working in developmental disabilities today knows about setting and meeting objectives which are measurable and timebound. Many variations of this concept are part of the training provided by our program. Since you must maintain performance standards and meet objectives every day of your professional lives, it is reasonable to expect you to do the same in an in-service training program designed to enhance your professional capabilities.

Admittedly, successful completion of the Management Training Program requires a sizeable commitment of time and effort. The two seminars and the site visit represent a combined total of 103 contact hours of training. Each of the eight home study assignments usually requires an additional 10 to 20 hours of effort. But the reward for this effort extends beyond the resulting improvement of your ability to manage. Upon successful completion of the program you will be awarded a certificate conferred by the University of Alabama in Birmingham. In addition, our program has been endorsed by the National Association of Superintendents of Public Residential Facilities for the Mentally Retarded. Efforts are now being made to have the certificate receive recognition by the appropriate personnel departments of state level mental retardation agencies where training is a contingency for promotion.

As a participant, you are now eligible to receive three to eight graduate credits for completing the program. To receive graduate credits, you must be accepted by the Graduate School of the University of Alabama in Birmingham or be enrolled in an accredited graduate program at another university. Graduate credits are obtained through one of three University of Alabama in Birmingham departments: School of Business, School of Education, or School of Community and Allied Health Resources. We hope eligibility for graduate credits will lead participants into a graduate-level program which includes a specialization in management of residential and community-based facilities for the mentally retarded.

If you think it would be a valuable or necessary addition to your professional credentials, you will also be eligible for continuing education credits. As stipulated by the Division of Continuing Medical Education, University of Alabama School of Medicine, eleven CEU's can be earned by completing the one year continuing education MTP: four CEU's for each of the two week-long seminars in Birmingham and three for the site visit.

And finally, perhaps the greatest reward realized by a Management Training Program participant is the lasting friendships that result from sharing problems and working with participants from many states—and the satisfaction in knowing that what has been gained from the program will result in better programs and services for retarded people.

For the most part, superintendents of facilities and state coordinators decide who is selected to participate in the Management Training Program. There are, no doubt, many individual factors which enter into this selection process. We understand this and have developed selection guidelines that may prove useful. These guidelines are the result of the consensus thinking of the MTP Advisory Committee and staff, with additional input from superintendents and state coordinators. They are not intended to cover every possible situation, nor must *every* guideline be used to judge a candidate for participation. In many cases one guideline will be sufficient to identify a person who would benefit from the program. The selection process should identify people who:

1. are career employees or new employees judged to have excellent career potential;
2. are employed in management positions or have acquired new or additional management responsibilities;
3. need management training to be eligible for promotion from a technical to a management position;
4. have expressed sincere motivation to upgrade their management skills;
5. understand the stringent requirements of the program and make the commitment to complete those requirements within the specified one-year period.

Once you have been selected as a participant, you are required:

130

1. to read the Management Training Program Overview before attending the first week seminar;
2. to record the dates of the first week seminar, final week seminar, and site visit on your personal calendar to avoid any scheduling conflicts;
3. to attend the two on-campus seminars and the site visit on the dates specified; (we realize that scheduling conflicts *do* happen; the training period for this program is one year; however, should conflicts arise, the training period can be extended an additional six months);
4. to complete the first three home study assignments before making your site visit;
5. to attend a half-day session on the Saturday morning of the site visit; (this session is used to complete Home Study Assignment #4 and the Site Visit Report);
6. to complete Home Study Assignments #5–8 before returning for the final week seminar; (these assignments are an essential introduction to the information presented in the final week);
7. to notify your superintendent or agency director and the director of the MTP if you wish to withdraw from the program;
8. to complete *all phases* of the program before receiving the certificate conferred by the University of Alabama in Birmingham;
9. to request from the director of the MTP the necessary forms and procedures for acquiring the three to eight graduate credits now available for participation in the MTP.

Guidelines for Acquiring Graduate Credit

The Management Training Program has been approved for three to eight graduate credits by the University of Alabama in Birmingham Schools of Business, Education, and Community and Allied Health Resources. You may acquire these credits in the following ways:

As a transient student. A transient student is one enrolled in a graduate program at another university. If you are in this category, obtain a Transient Application from the University of Alabama in Birmingham Graduate Office. Complete the first portion of the form and have your university graduate official complete and sign the middle portion stating that you are a graduate student in good standing. Your school officials will mail the form to the Graduate School, University of Alabama in Birmingham. The last portion of the form requires the UAB Graduate Dean's signature and serves as the Admission Slip which allows you to register. The Graduate School will furnish you a copy of the completed form. YOU MUST BE FULLY ADMITTED TO GRADUATE SCHOOL BEFORE ATTEMPTING TO REGISTER.

As a student not actively enrolled in another graduate program. If you are *not* actively enrolled in a graduate program, you must apply to the University of Alabama in Birmingham as a new student. You will need to complete the UAB Graduate Application Form and return it with three letters of reference and two official transcripts from each of the colleges you attended to obtain your Baccalaureate Degree. In addition, you must take one of the following tests for admission to graduate study:

1. The Graduate Record Exam (GRE). The aptitude portion is required; minimum score of 1,000 for admission in good standing.
2. The Miller Analogies Test (MAT). Minimum score of 35 is needed for admission to School of Education; minimum score of 50 is needed for admission to SCAHR.
3. The Graduate Management Admissions Test (GMAT). For applicants entering the School of Business MBA Program; minimum score of 450 is required.
4. National Teachers Examination (NTE). Minimum score of 600 common, 1,200 composite, for admission in good standing.

The specific examinations required by the schools offering the Management Training Program course are:

Area of Study	Entrance Exam
Education	GRE or NTE or MAT
Business Administration	GMAT
Hospital Administration	GMAT or GRE or MAT

Instate Tuition is $225 per quarter (maximum), or $34 per credit hour. Out-of-State Tuition is $450 per quarter (maximum), or $68 per credit hour. For Graduate Application Forms and Graduate School Bulletins, write to:

> Dean of the Graduate School
> University of Alabama in Birmingham
> University Station
> 1045 9th Avenue, South
> Birmingham, Alabama 35294

Staff and Faculty

The instructional input for the two week-long seminars of the Management Training Program is provided by the six member Program staff and the excellent faculty available from the School of Business, School of Education, and School of Community and Allied Health Resources at the University of Alabama in Birmingham. Additional faculty and consultants have been recruited from outside the University to provide expertise where needed.

Management Training Program Curriculum Outline

I. **First Week Seminar.** Participants begin the one year program with this seminar at the Center for Developmental and Learning Disorders in Birmingham. This is the participant's introduction to the instructional content of the program. These topics make up the first week curriculum:

A. Managerial Grid Theory
   1. Topic Description
      a) "Styles of Management Inventory" is administered to participants.
      b) Inventory results are interpreted in terms of the characteristics of five basic styles of management on the Blake and Mouton "Managerial Grid."
   2. Purpose
      a) To have participants identify characteristics of five basic management styles and their influence on an organization.
      b) To have participants understand their own predominant management style and their backup style as indicated by the "Styles of Management Inventory."
      c) To have participants understand the advantages of 9/9 team approach to management.

B. Decision Making
   1. Topic Description
      a) Participants analyze and evaluate their own decision-making process.
      b) "Griffith's Six Steps in Decision Making" is presented as a logical, viable process.
   2. Purpose
      a) To provide a logical process for recognizing and defining a problem.
      b) To provide a logical process for analyzing and evaluating solutions to problems.
      c) To provide a logical process for selecting a preferred solution to a problem.

C. Basic Concepts of Management
   1. Topic Description
      a) Management is presented as a profession and defined as "getting things done through other people."

    b) The basic components of management are:
       (1) Planning
       (2) Organizing
       (3) Controlling
       (4) Motivating
       (5) Communicating
    c) There are four essentials of organization:
       (1) Authority
       (2) Reportability
       (3) Responsibility
       (4) Accountability
2. Purpose
    a) To have participants realize that management is a professional responsibility apart from whatever other technical expertise they may have.
    b) To provide participants with the basic aspects of management and a definition of their role as a manager within an organization.

D. Organization Climates
  1. Topic Description
    a) Participants are presented with the universal conflict between the demands of the internal organization and the external environment which influences the organization.
    b) Participants are provided with a philosophy and some strategies for dealing with and controlling the change caused by external influence.
  2. Purpose
    a) To describe how externalities influence an organization.
    b) To change that management thinking which pleads an inability to control the influence of externalities.

c) To provide a systematic process for:
    (1) Dealing with externalities
    (2) Adapting effectively to change caused by externalities

E. Labor Relations
  1. Topic Description
    a) Participants are provided with a topic outline which delineates the impact of employee organization on management and management style.
    b) Participants are involved in a lecture/discussion analyzing the positive and negative effects of unionization on an organization serving the mentally retarded.
  2. Purpose
    a) To analyze the effects of unionization of an organization.
    b) To critique employee relations in terms of why employees join unions.
    c) To review the basic goals and objectives of labor organizations.
    d) To present the mechanics of collective bargaining.
    e) To present examples of the effects of labor organization and collective bargaining on Blake and Mouton's five basic styles of management.

F. Interpersonal Relationships: Communications and Motivation
  1. Topic Description
    a) Analyzes communication theory and its application to managing an organization.
    b) Analyzes what motivates employees to perform or not perform their function with an organization.
    c) Analyzes the way communication theory relates to motivation of employees.

2. Purpose
   a) To have participants evaluate their own organizations in terms of the communications and motivation theories presented.
   b) Have participants relate these theories to five basic styles of management (Managerial Grid Theory).

G. Management Organization and Job Descriptions
   1. Topic Description
      a) Provides a basic definition of and rationale for traditional organization structure.
      b) Presents nine basic principles of organization as defined by the American Management Association:
         (1) Objective
         (2) Coordination
         (3) Authority
         (4) Responsibility
         (5) Accountability
         (6) Definition
         (7) Span of control
         (8) Unity of command
         (9) Delegation
      c) Presents a logic for creating specific job descriptions for all people who function within an organization.
      d) Presents five essential elements needed in a job description:
         (1) Job function
         (2) Authority
         (3) Responsibility
         (4) Reportability
         (5) Accountability
   2. Purpose
      a) To give participants the basic premise on which the whole concept of management is based.

b) To provide an informational base from which participants can evaluate their own organization and their functions within that organization.

c) To encourage participants to see the value that clearly defined job descriptions have in organization structure and function.

d) To provide participants with the essentials and format for writing well-defined job descriptions.

H. Legal Aspects of Mental Retardation
1. Topic Description
   a) Provides an analysis of important legal cases.
      (1) Right to treatment
      (2) Right to education
      (3) Right to compensation
   b) Provides a forum for discussion of the legal principles involved.
   c) Looks at the ethical and moral questions now being raised in the area of:
      (1) Commitment
      (2) Guardianship
      (3) Intervention of the courts in the administrative process
2. Purpose
   a) To inform and sensitize participants on the issues of both legal and individual rights of the mentally retarded.
   b) To have participants understand their professional responsibility to uphold and promote the rights of the retarded.
   c) To encourage participants to analyze their profession for practices that abridge the rights of those persons in their care.

I. Organization Development
1. Topic Description

138

a) Differentiates between process and content in the accomplishment of organizational objectives.
   (1) Process—how a person goes about doing *something*.
   (2) Content—the *something* that is actually done.
b) Defines and uses structured experiences.
   (1) Short, goal-oriented tasks designed to examine participants' behavior (process) that is manifested in order to accomplish the task.
   (2) Designed to examine *how* a participant gets things done.
c) Relates the observed individual behaviors and interpersonal relationships by analogy to interactions in organizations and their effect on organizations.

2. Structured Experiences
   a) Broken Squares Puzzles
      (1) Description: A group of five people attempts to cooperate in putting together five broken squares without speaking to each other.
      (2) Purpose
         (a) To analyze cooperation in solving a group problem.
         (b) To sensitize participants to behaviors that contribute toward or obstruct the solving of a group problem.
   b) Goal Clarity
      (1) Description: Participant groups are given two written statements of goals to achieve. One is quite specific; the other is hopelessly vague and unobtainable. Observers record group behavior as they work toward meeting each goal.

(2) Purpose
   (a) To establish the importance of well-defined goals.
   (b) To dramatize the difference in group behavior when a goal is vague and unobtainable as opposed to a goal which is clear and obtainable.

c) NASA Exercise
   (1) Description: Individually, and then in groups, participants must rank in order of priority a list of fifteen survival items they would need if stranded on the moon.
   (2) Purpose
      (a) To evaluate the results of individual decisions.
      (b) To evaluate the results of group concensus decisions.
      (c) Compare individual decisions to group decisions to illustrate the value of group consensus judgement.

d) Transatlantic Flight
   (1) Description: Individually, and then in groups, participants decide which persons from a descriptive list they are given will be thrown off an airplane to prevent it from crashing.
   (2) Purpose: To illustrate how bias affects both individual and group decisions.

e) Personal Goals
   (1) Description: Participants write a list of professional goals for themselves and put them in a self-addressed envelope. They are mailed to each participant in thirty days.

(2) Purpose: To provide participants with a self-evaluation of their goals and achievements.

J. Simulation—Instructional activities are brought together throughout the week by the utilization of the *Shannon State School and Hospital Simulation Training Materials*, which are specifically designed to link theory and practice for management personnel employed in facilities serving the mentally retarded. Simulation includes the following:
1. Video-Taped Personal Encounters
   a) *Kennedy/Roble: Participant, as superintendent, encounters Roble, the personnel officer, who is arrogant and powerful within the organization.
   b) Kennedy/Marek: Participant, as superintendent, encounters Marek, the local union president, over labor problems and resident peonage.
   c) Kennedy/Shrister: Participant, as superintendent, encounters Shrister, soft drink salesman interested in promoting his product through institution publicity.
   d) Kennedy/Kelly: Participant, as superintendent, encounters a part-time recreation worker who reports a case of resident abuse.
   e) Kennedy/Jacobson: Participant, as superintendent, encounters Mrs. Jacobson, the local ARC president, who seeks a number of commitments.
   f) Kennedy/Coleman: Participant, as superintendent, encounters the director of Shannon's department of education and train-

* Val Kennedy is the name of the Superintendent of Shannon State School and Hospital. This is the name and position assumed by participants in the Simulator.

141

ing, who is questioning the logic of a past practice.

g) Swimming Pool Encounter: Participant, as superintendent, presides over a meeting of his staff and community officials. At stake are twenty season tickets bought so Shannon residents can use the community swimming pool.

2. Telephone Calls (received by participant, as superintendent, during personal encounters).

a) Mrs. Regina—Calls to complain about Roble, the personnel director, and hiring practices at Shannon.

b) Anonymous caller—Calls to warn superintendent that his director of nursing, Ramona Linck, is leading a community movement to keep facility residents out of the community swimming pool.

c) Mrs. Short—Calls from a flower shop to see if Kennedy wishes to continue a standing order of flowers for the former superintendent's secretary.

d) Mrs. Wilmar—Calls to request more information on evidence of physical abuse to her child, a resident.

e) William Kerr—As community pool director, he claims trickery in purchase of season tickets and wants them back.

3. In-Basket Items (participants read, discuss, and expedite these each day).

a) Set #1

(1) Three-page letter from Commissioner

(2) Telephone message from secretary

(3) Welcome letter from ARC President

(4) Personnel director's memo on walk-in applicants

(5) Irate letter from a resident's parents

b) Set #2
   (1) Union president's letter on resident labor
   (2) Parent letter disputing son's vocational placement
   (3) Union representative requesting permission to post notices
   (4) Nurse's letter of resignation
   (5) Fire Chief's letter on fire regulations
c) Set #3
   (1) Letter from computer company selling education program
   (2) Anonymous letter on pool issue
   (3) Telephone message about missing resident
   (4) Letter from parents requesting commitment of their child
   (5) Letter from university outlining research project
d) Set #4
   (1) Parent letter requesting special diet for child
   (2) Parent letter requesting religious confirmation
   (3) Parent letter seeking progress report on son
   (4) Nurse's memo reporting alleged resident abuse
   (5) Mayor's letter of invitation to town council meeting
e) Set #5
   (1) Telephone message from sheriff about resident
   (2) Regional commissioner's letter vetoing staff member's leave
   (3) Memo requesting change in procedure manual

        (4) Memo from nurse reporting stolen drugs
        (5) Telephone message reporting a stranger with camera
        (6) Letter from community complaining about institution's appearance

II. **Home Study Assignments.** These eight assignments are given to participants at the end of the first week seminar. The assignments are to be completed and mailed to MTP faculty for evaluation. All assignments must be completed before participant returns for the final week seminar.

  A. Assignments related to the first week seminar

      1. Assignment #1: Multiple Choice Exercise—seventy-five questions, open book exercise intended to reinforce the information taught during the first week seminar.

      2. Assignment #2: Employee Appraisal System Manual—two position descriptions with standards of performance are written by participants applicable to their work situation.

      3. Assignment #3: Labor Relations—the development of a contingency plan for a union-precipitated emergency, and an explanation of the grievance procedures used at the participant's institution.

  B. Assignment related to the site visit midway through the training year.

      1. Assignment #4: Site Visit Analysis—an objective compilation of the participant's observations of the guest facility's organizational structure, procedures, and programs.

      2. Report to facility: Includes information from all site visit participants *exclusive* of affective judgements of individual personalities and performance. Report is *not* an evaluation or assessment of facility's program effectiveness.

C. Assignments introducing the content taught in final week seminar.
   1. Assignment #5: Programmed Evaluation Review Technique (PERT)—use of two programmed instruction books and an application of PERT to a real situation in each participant's own facility.
   2. Assignment #6: Principles of Public Relations —emphasis on the development of an effective program to communicate information both within an organization and to the world around it.
   3. Assignment #7: Issues, Trends, Problems, and Innovations in Mental Retardation—a short answer essay format requiring an awareness of a variety of topics considered essential in the management of a mental retardation facility.
   4. Assignment #8: Budgeting and Accounting— two programmed instruction texts which emphasize basic budgeting and accounting principles for participants with no previous experience in these areas.

D. Alternate Assignments which may be substituted when one or more of the required assignments are of limited value to participants in their work situations.
   1. Alternate Assignment #1: *Principles of Management*—a programmed instruction text which provides an overview of the basic management concepts taught throughout the program.
   2. Alternate Assignment #2: Multiple Choice Learning Exercise—100 questions introducing the instructional content of and providing a common frame of reference for the final week seminar.
   3. Alternate Assignment #3: *Introduction to Data Processing*—a programmed instruction text

which provides information on computerized information and dissemination.

III. **Site Visit.** Conducted midway through the participant's training year.
    A. Description
        1. Group of participants meet at a site visit facility chosen by the MTP and spend three days observing and discussing the facility's organization and programs. This interaction occurs between staff, participants, and the participant counterparts at the site visit facility.
        2. Each participant completes Home Study Assignment #4. This requires participants to:
            a) Analyze site visit facility's organization in terms of:
                (1) Lines of authority
                    (a) Formal
                    (b) Informal
                (2) Lines of communication and communication barriers
            b) Revise and hopefully improve the guest facility's organization chart.
            c) Interview position counterparts at the facility.
            d) Identify and discuss facility's various systems, procedures, programs, etc.
            e) Discuss facility programs relevant to their own needs.
            f) Create positive inter-institution relations among management personnel.
    B. Purpose
        1. To increase participant knowledge regarding institution and community-based:
            a) Organization
            b) Operating procedures
            c) Programming

d) Service delivery systems
2. To provide participants with information which will result in improvement, modification, or development of programs at their own facilities.

IV. **Final Week Seminar.** At the end of the training year, the participant returns to the Center for Developmental and Learning Disorders in Birmingham for the final week seminar. These topics make up the final week curriculum:

A. Budget Preparation
   1. Topic Description
      a) Identifies and analyzes a budget as a quantitative expression of a plan of action to meet organization objectives.
      b) Presents budgets as an aid to coordination and control of organizational plan of action.
      c) Studies the major types of budgets and the budgeting process in conjunction with the participant's knowledge of information from Home Study Assignment #7.
   2. Purpose
      a) To give participants a basic understanding of budgeting and the budgeting process.
      b) To give participants a working knowledge of budgeting terminology.
      c) To emphasize to participants the value of budget information in coordinating and controlling organization plans.
      d) To analyze the effect of a superintendent's management style on the formulation and implementation of a budget.

B. Program Evaluation Review Technique
   1. Topic Description
      a) PERT is a management technique that

facilitates the implementation of a management objective or project in terms of:
- (1) Time
- (2) Cost (resources)
- (3) Performance

   b) Application of the PERT methodology is made to management planning and control functions.

   c) Special emphasis is given to relating PERT to specific managerial problems and objectives.

  2. Purpose

   a) To provide participants with a basic understanding of PERT methodology.

   b) To have participants apply PERT methodology to a specific management objective to see its value as an aid in planning and controlling.

C. Computerized Data Processing

  1. Topic Description

   a) Review and analysis of the value of data processing as applied to planning and organizing the business and support services of mental retardation facilities.

   b) Presents information on how computer-based data processing can be applied to resident programming in mental retardation facilities.

  2. Purpose

   a) To present information on the role computerized data processing plays in each of these managerial functions:
- (1) Planning
- (2) Organizing
- (3) Controlling
- (4) Communicating
- (5) Motivating

b) To describe the step-by-step procedure for applying computerized data processing to:
   (1) Individualized resident habilitation plans
   (2) Medical care for residents
c) Present examples of applications of computerized data processing that have failed in the context of a mental retardation facility.

D. Fundamentals of Financial Accounting
   1. Topic Description
      a) Basic information on financial accounting is presented in terms that a person with little or no background in accounting can understand.
         (1) Information is referenced to participant's knowledge gained from Home Study Assignment #7.
         (2) A knowledge of accounting must precede a later component of the curriculum on budgeting.
      b) Participant analyzes and discusses the concept that an accountant exists in an organization to provide management with the financial information needed to meet program objectives.
   2. Purpose
      a) To provide nonaccountant type managers with a basic understanding of accounting techniques, procedures, and terminology.
      b) To enable participants to interpret a simple financial statement.
      c) To analyze and discuss the fact that accounting procedures and financial statements are tools of control for managers.

E. Employee Counseling and Performance Appraisal

1. Topic Description
   a) This is a continuation of the presentation of a total organization system begun with the component on Management Organization and Job Descriptions.
   b) Provides a system and format for developing effective employee appraisals of performance using objective standards of performance.
   c) Compares this design for creating and implementing an employee performance appraisal system with the system currently being used by their own organizations.
   d) Provides a comprehensive model of the system as used by the state employees of the state of Minnesota.
2. Purpose
   a) To have participants analyze the virtues and faults of this employee appraisal system in comparison with the system currently used by their institution organizations.
   b) To have participants understand the employee appraisal should be directed to positive development of an employee's abilities and should not be used as a yearly punitive measure related to promotion and salary increases.
   c) To give participants four basic criteria for writing performance standards.
   d) To give participants the four steps in the employee appraisal process.

F. Public Relations: Principles and Practices
   1. Topic Description
      a) Part One deals with the Internal communication of information within an organization. Relation is made to a book,

Hospital PR . . . by Objectives by Joe G. Hochderffer, and Home Study Assignment #4.

  b) Part Two uses a video-taped simulation encounter as a vehicle to discuss ways of communicating information about the organization to the external public. Reference is also made to Home Study Assignment #4.

  2. Purpose
  a) To give participants an understanding of the importance and scope of public relations and information dissemination.
  b) To point out that everyone employed by the institution is a public relations practitioner for that organization.
  c) To point out that there are really no specific boundaries or rules to follow in practicing public relations.

G. Alternatives to Institutionalization
  1. Topic Description
  a) The Program provides a guest lecturer on deinstitutionalization and/or institutional reform.
  b) Discussion on finance, legislation, and programs are included with these seminar components.
  c) Discussion and analysis is encouraged on creating and administrating a system of community-based facilities.
  d) A system is presented which offers a system of evolving from institutional incarceration of the mentally retarded to the least restrictive alternative of community placement of some sort.

  2. Purpose
  a) To provide the participants with as broad and comprehensive an overview as possible

of the current trend in MR toward de-institutionalization and institutional reform.
b) To share with participants various views and solutions of professionals working in mental retardation.
c) To give participants a forum to question and discuss current issues and trends in mental retardation.

H. Effective Written Communications
   1. Topic Description
      a) Presents the rudiments of clear written communications in reference to the categories of:
         (1) Letters
         (2) Memos
         (3) Reports
      b) Includes a structured experience which emphasizes the problem of communicating effectively via the written word.
      c) Asks four questions about any written communication which summarizes the essential components of all good writing.
         (1) Is the written communication *clear*?
         (2) Is the written communication *concise*?
         (3) Is the written communication *conversational*?
         (4) Is the written communication *correct*?
      d) Provides a number of handouts and a book, *The Elements of Style* by William Strunk, Jr., which serve as writing references for the participants.
   2. Purpose
      a) To provide participants with advice on particular writing problems relative to their professional responsibilities.

b) To provide participants with material and information which will help them produce better written communications in terms of clarity, conciseness, and correctness.

I. Organization Development
  1. Topic Description (see Part I, Section I)
  2. Structured Experiences
    a) Brainstorming
      (1) Description: Participants are asked individually and then in groups to list all the uses they would find for a belt buckle if they were stranded on a desert island.
      (2) Purpose
        (a) To relax participants and get their minds working.
        (b) To point out that the suggestions of others should not be denigrated.
    b) Choosing-a-Color and Leadership Characteristics
      (1) Description: The instructor describes various roles the participants in a group meeting take on. Roles are assigned to all members of the group, and the group is given a problem to solve. Post-exercise discussion has the group identify all the assigned roles of the individuals.
      (2) Purpose
        (a) To explore the behaviors of various roles and their effect on the group process.
        (b) To identify leadership within the group (two leader roles are assigned) and analyze the effects of shared leadership.
    c) World Bank

(1) Description: After each contributes $2.00 to the World Bank, participants are divided into two groups. The two groups are separated and given a task to perform at given time intervals. They can negotiate with each other between time intervals upon request and consent. If the two groups trust each other and cooperate, each participant's $2.00 is returned. If not, they lose all or a portion of their money to the World Bank.

(2) Purpose
    (a) To see the results of group goal displacement.
    (b) To see the effects of high or low trust levels on interaction between individuals and groups.
    (c) To compare the results of this structured experience to the relations between departments or divisions of an organization.

d) Win-As-Much-As-You-Can
(1) Description: Participants are paired off and given the impression that, if they play the game properly, they can win a great deal of money, at the expense of the other pairs. However, if they read the instructions carefully, they find that by cooperating with the other pairs, everyone can win a reasonable amount. If pairs decide to go it alone, they gamble with the possibility of winning or losing a great deal.

(2) Purpose
    (a) To illustrate the value to all of cooperating with everyone.

        (b) To illustrate the effects of high or low trust levels on group interaction and goal attainment.

        (c) To compare this experience to inter-departmental cooperation or lack of it in an organization.

  e) Lutts and Mipps

    (1) Description: Participants are given twenty-six information cards. They pretend that lutts and mipps represent a new way of measuring distance and that dars, wors, and mirs represent a new way of measuring time. A man drives from Town A, through Town B and Town C, to Town D. The group's task is to determine how many wors the entire trip took. No formal leader is chosen.

    (2) Purpose

        (a) To analyze the sharing of information in a task-oriented group.

        (b) To emphasize the value of cooperation in group problem solving.

        (c) To observe the emergence of leadership behavior in group problem solving.

J. Simulation: Final week instructional activities are tied together throughout the week by the utilization of the *Shannon State School and Hospital Simulator* which is specifically designed to link theory and practice for management personnel employed in facilities serving the mentally retarded. Simulation includes the following:

1. Video-Taped Personal Encounters

  a) Kennedy/Shaffer: Participant, as superintendent, encounters Shaffer, from Central

Office, who pressures for implementation of Central Office workshops against resistance from institution Training and Education Department.

b) Kennedy/Brace: Participant, as superintendent, encounters Brace, Director of Volunteer Services, who seeks decision on firing of staff member alleged to be drinking on the job.

c) Kennedy/Poole: Participant, as superintendent, encounters Poole, administrative secretary, who wants to resign immediately because of overwhelming personal problems.

d) Kennedy/Benish/Jacobson: Participant, as superintendent, encounters Benish, a CBS reporter, and Jacobson, local ARC President, in his office just as he receives a telephone call reporting the fatal stabbing of a resident (used in conjunction with the Public Relations component of the seminar).

e) Kennedy/Dr. Greene: Participant, as superintendent, encounters Dr. Greene, Director of Medical Services, who complains about other institution departments' resisting his advice and orders and threatens to resign.

f) Kennedy/Coleman: Participant, as superintendent, encounters Coleman, Director of Training and Education, who presents his reasons for resisting the Central Office and its workshops.

g) Kennedy/Houston: Participant, as superintendent, encounters Houston as a candidate to be interviewed for position of administrative secretary.

156

h) Kennedy/Longwith: Participant, as superintendent, encounters Longwith, Regional Director and Kennedy's immediate superordinate, who wants placement of his two staff members, who are problems, on the Shannon staff.

i) Mickey Ranier Show: Participant, as superintendent, appears on a local TV show. He is questioned by the host and phone calls from the community on current issues and trends in mental retardation.

j) Staff Meeting: Participant, as superintendent, conducts a meeting of several staff members from different departments and Shaffer, from Central Office, in an effort to resolve the conflict over Central Office workshops.

2. Telephone Calls received by participant, as superintendent, during the personal encounters.

a) Passerby: Calls from town to report a resident who has missed his bus back to the institution.

b) Helen Baxley (A Volunteer Worker): Calls from Camp Ken-A-Wood, twenty-five miles from institution, to report twenty-six residents are ill with food poisoning.

c) Mickey Ranier: Calls to invite Kennedy to appear on a TV interview show on Friday morning. Subject will be "Current Issues and Trends in MR."

d) Dr. Greene: Calls to report the fatal stabbing of a resident and to seek advice on what to do.

e) Jim Roble: Calls for decision regarding a security guard who suffered a stroke and can't do his job. Problem is whether to carry him on the payroll or release him.

f) Senator Watkins: Calls at the request of a constituent to inquire about a resident scheduled for release from the institution.

g) FBI Agent Pyle: Calls as part of an investigation into a threatening letter to the president written, signed, and sent by an institution resident.

h) Commissioner Webster: Calls to request an immediate and complete report on the resident stabbing.

3. In-Basket Items (participants read, discuss, and expedite these each day).

a) Set #1

(1) Letter from Commissioner requesting change in institution organization and philosophy.

(2) Letter from a family requesting to visit a resident who is not related to them.

(3) Memo from Coleman complaining about medical influence on staff meetings.

(4) Memo from union president asking for information on suspension of a member.

(5) Memo from accountant about surplus of unspent grant funds.

b) Set #2

(1) Memo from Care and Treatment Department complaining of medical interference in resident exercise.

(2) Letter of application from a foreign-born and educated M.D.

(3) Complimentary letter from resident's parents on institution programs.

(4) Memo from institution concerning excessive milk production.

(5) Memo from supervisor complaining about merit-rating changes on one of his men.

c) Set #3

(1) Mickey Ranier letter with TV show questions.

(2) Memo from Roble and resume of candidate for secretary position.

(3) Memo from Psychology Department affirming the value of Central Office workshop.

(4) Regional Director's memo on establishing institution research departments.

(5) Letter from family whose son died at institution.

(6) Letter requesting Kennedy address the county American Medical Association.

d) Set #4

(1) Letter from parents requesting chiropractic treatment for son.

(2) Telephone call from nurse about employee-rating disagreement.

(3) Memo from Psychological Services about institution procedures manual.

(4) Memo from Business Manager asking what department gets priority on a new truck.

(5) Memo from nurse about poor condition of the morgue.

e) Set #5

(1) Telephone message requesting appointment to demonstrate fertilizer.

(2) Memo from Business Manager about dispersal of unused equipment.

(3) Memo from Food Service complaining about guests for lunch.

(4) Memo complaining about recruiting for LPN Association during working hours.

(5) Letter from parents requesting daughter be transferred to community facility.

APPENDIX E

Management Issues Relevant to
Mental Health Continuing Education

*Western Interstate Commission
on Higher Education Conference
June, 1975*

If mental health organizations import people, resources, information, and theory from the environment and transform them into outputs with "added value," this raises important issues:

I. How are society's expectations changing with regard to mental health?
    1. The custodian, healer, preventer issue.
    2. The accountability issue
       a) What you must do must be done efficiently.
       b) Accountable to whom?
    3. Human rights
       a) The rights of patients, including the right to treatment.
       b) Equity in terms of who is served.
       c) Equity in terms of who makes policy and who governs.
       d) Equity in employment.

II. How are new technologies likely to change the role of mental health organizations?
    4. Further advances in pharmacology, molecular biology, genetics, behavior modification, bio-feedback, etc.
    5. Advances in "allied" organizations which reduce social stress by improving the economy and employment, social security, physical health, etc.

III. How will new sources of funding affect mental health organizations?
    6. Changing from a grants economy to a world of third-party payments.
    7. Multiple source funding and the energy required for multiple source lobbying and the internal juggling of multiple demands and regulations from multiple funders.

IV. How will new social expectations, technologies, and funding sources affect:

8. The mission of mental health organizations, long-range purposes, and goals?

9. The types of human skills required—and ways for sorting, training, credentialing, updating, and adapting these varieties of skills?

10. The types of organizational arrangements necessary to deal with these new expectations?

   a) Maintaining a useable identity in an umbrella agency.

   b) Linkages, consortia, alliances, coalitions, and vendettas with allies and competitors.

   c) Consumer inputs, consumer advocacy, client feedback.

V. What types of managerial arrangements are necessary to:

11. Monitor changes in social expectations and technological advances?

12. Live with a dynamic, flexible, polymorphic goal structure?

13. Set a framework and useable process for determining priorities?

14. Balance rational data and logical processes with political realities?

15. Develop a typology of needed leadership styles, select and develop leaders and middle managers?

16. Determine what types of decision making are required, and which types may justifiably absorb major energies and long-term focus?

17. Set up monitoring systems which assure efficient use of resources?

18. Set up monitoring systems which satisfy "resource providers?"

19. Set up monitoring systems which promote staff growth and the development of useable knowledge —including "scientific" or theory knowledge?

VI. How does a mental health system respond to the diverse

needs of a society of plural cultures, changing values, unpredictable sources of stress?

    20. Can racism be replaced with services useable by all portions of society?

VII. What are the implications of management problems for the continuing education practitioners in terms of:

    21. Roles, role blurring, role conflict, role change—for all disciplines?

    22. Continuing Education for individual career development versus organizational/system needs?

    23. Knowledge updating versus attitudinal change versus organizational development?